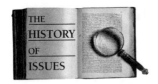

Public Health

Other Books in the History of Issues Series:

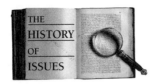

THE
HISTORY
OF
ISSUES

Public Health

Adriane Ruggiero, Book Editor

GREENHAVEN PRESS

An imprint of Thomson Gale, a part of The Thomson Corporation

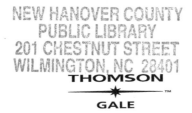

THOMSON
━━━✦━━━ ™
GALE

Detroit • New York • San Francisco • New Haven, Conn. • Waterville, Maine • London

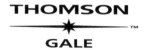

Christine Nasso, *Publisher*
Elizabeth Des Chenes, *Managing Editor*

© 2007 The Gale Group.

Star logo is a trademark and Gale and Greenhaven Press are registered trademarks used herein under license.

For more information, contact: Greenhaven Press
27500 Drake Rd.
Farmington Hills, MI 48331-3535
Or you can visit our Internet site at http://www.gale.com

Cover photograph © Christopher J. Morris/Corbis

ISBN-13: 978-0-7377-3846-9
ISBN-10: 0-7377-3846-4

2007932782

Contents

Chapter 1: The Origins of Public Health

Chapter 2: Public Health in the United States Through Mid-Twentieth Century

Chapter 3: Public Health in the United States, Mid-Twentieth Century to the Present

Chapter 4: Global Public Health Challenges for the Future

Foreword

In the 1940s, at the height of the Holocaust, Jews struggled to create a nation of their own in Palestine, a region of the Middle East that at the time was controlled by Britain. The British had placed limits on Jewish immigration to Palestine, hampering efforts to provide refuge to Jews fleeing the Holocaust. In response to this and other British policies, an underground Jewish resistance group called Irgun began carrying out terrorist attacks against British targets in Palestine, including immigration, intelligence, and police offices. Most famously, the group bombed the King David Hotel in Jerusalem, the site of a British military headquarters. Although the British were warned well in advance of the attack, they failed to evacuate the building. As a result, ninety-one people were killed (including fifteen Jews) and forty-five were injured.

Early in the twentieth century, Ireland, which had long been under British rule, was split into two countries. The south, populated mostly by Catholics, eventually achieved independence and became the Republic of Ireland. Northern Ireland, mostly Protestant, remained under British control. Catholics in both the north and south opposed British control of the north, and the Irish Republican Army (IRA) sought unification of Ireland as an independent nation. In 1969, the IRA split into two factions. A new radical wing, the Provisional IRA, was created and soon undertook numerous terrorist bombings and killings throughout Northern Ireland, the Republic of Ireland, and even in England. One of its most notorious attacks was the 1974 bombing of a Birmingham, England, bar that killed nineteen people.

In the mid-1990s, an Islamic terrorist group called al Qaeda began carrying out terrorist attacks against American targets overseas. In communications to the media, the organization listed several complaints against the United States. It generally opposed all U.S. involvement and presence in the Middle East. It particularly objected to the presence of U.S. troops in Saudi Arabia, which is the home of several Islamic holy sites. And it strongly condemned the United States for supporting the nation of Israel, which it claimed was an oppressor of Muslims. In 1998 al Qaeda's leaders issued a fatwa (a religious legal statement) calling for Muslims to kill Americans. Al Qaeda acted on this order many times—most memorably on September 11, 2001, when it attacked the World Trade Center and the Pentagon, killing nearly three thousand people.

These three groups—Irgun, the Provisional IRA, and al Qaeda—have achieved varied results. Irgun's terror campaign contributed to Britain's decision to pull out of Palestine and to support the creation of Israel in 1948. The Provisional IRA's tactics kept pressure on the British, but they also alienated many would-be supporters of independence for Northern Ireland. Al Qaeda's attacks provoked a strong U.S. military response but did not lessen America's involvement in the Middle East nor weaken its support of Israel. Despite these different results, the means and goals of these groups were similar. Although they emerged in different parts of the world during different eras and in support of different causes, all three had one thing in common: They all used clandestine violence to undermine a government they deemed oppressive or illegitimate.

The destruction of oppressive governments is not the only goal of terrorism. For example, terror is also used to minimize dissent in totalitarian regimes and to promote extreme ideologies. However, throughout history the motivations of terrorists have been remarkably similar, proving the old adage that "the more things change, the more they remain the same." Arguments for and against terrorism thus boil down to the same set of universal arguments regardless of the age: Some argue that terrorism is justified to change (or, in the case of state terror, to maintain) the prevailing political order; others respond that terrorism is inhumane and unacceptable under any circumstances. These basic views transcend time and place.

Similar fundamental arguments apply to other controversial social issues. For instance, arguments over the death penalty have always featured competing views of justice. Scholars cite biblical texts to claim that a person who takes a life must forfeit his or her life, while others cite religious doctrine to support their view that only God can take a human life. These arguments have remained essentially the same throughout the centuries. Likewise, the debate over euthanasia has persisted throughout the history of Western civilization. Supporters argue that it is compassionate to end the suffering of the dying by hastening their impending death; opponents insist that it is society's duty to make the dying as comfortable as possible as death takes its natural course.

Greenhaven Press's The History of Issues series illustrates this constancy of arguments surrounding major social issues. Each volume in the series focuses on one issue—including terrorism, the death penalty, and euthanasia—and examines how the debates have both evolved and remained essentially the same over the years. Primary documents such as newspaper articles, speeches, and government reports illuminate historical developments and offer perspectives from throughout history. Secondary sources provide overviews and commentaries from a more contemporary perspective. An introduction begins each anthology and supplies essential context and background. An annotated table of contents, chronology, and index allow for easy reference, and a bibliography and list of organizations to contact point to additional sources of information on the book's topic. With these features, The History of Issues series permits readers to glimpse both the historical and contemporary dimensions of humanity's most pressing and controversial social issues.

Introduction

Childhood obesity is one of the most pressing public health issues in the United States in the twenty-first century and threatens to become an all-out crisis. According to the Alliance for a Healthier Generation, about 25 million kids ages two to nineteen in the United States are overweight or at risk of becoming overweight. That is nearly one of every three kids. The increase in the number of children who are overweight was noticed about twenty to thirty years ago and is now epidemic in the United States. Obesity is seen in children and teens of all races and both genders. Obese children are at risk for developing such chronic diseases as type 2 diabetes, high blood pressure, high cholesterol levels, and depression. The issue has evolved over the years from a discussion by pediatricians and some educators to an all-out dialogue by the medical community, schools, government leaders, and healthcare advocates. The consensus reached is that if nothing is done to correct the problem, overweight boys and girls living in the early 2000s will have lower life expectancies than their parents.

Not Just in the Genes

For a while it was generally believed that obesity was linked to genetics and that the chubby boy or girl was destined to become a fat man or woman. There was a certain degree of passivity among doctors with regard to helping obese people lose weight. For the most part doctors prescribed diets and left individuals to their own devices to shed the necessary pounds. More often than not, people wanted to lose weight for cosmetic reasons and were unaware of the link between obesity and health. Sadly, many of these dieters failed to keep the weight off in the long run and became resigned to being fat for life. When more and more children were diagnosed with obesity, however, other hypotheses about the disease came into play. In recent years health professionals and others have pointed to several key factors contributing to obesity. These include the increased popularity of fast food as the primary meal eaten by many families, the growing size of portions served by many fast-food restaurants, the overuse of processed foods in American households, a sedentary lifestyle, and the abuse of food to mask a variety of psychological issues. Another factor much discussed by health-care commentators is the present generation's desire for instant gratification as part of a societal attitude toward food and other objects. Thus arose the nickname of "fast-food generation."

Ending the Fast-Food Attitude

What is the solution to the problem of childhood obesity? Are kids too concerned about their weight because they fear being teased or bullied? In one of the richest nations in the world do too many children lack access to fresh and healthful foods? Are parents so busy that they cannot pay attention to what their children eat? Are children capable of making healthful food choices on their own? What are the best strategies for preventing obesity? What treatments work over a long time? Researchers are trying to answer these and many other questions.

Changing eating habits in the family is fundamental in the fight against childhood obesity, say many experts. In its guidelines for parents, the American Obesity Association (AOA) urges mothers and fathers to take charge of family eating habits. The AOA suggests that families limit the number of times they eat out at fast-food restaurants, establish regular hours for meals, and provide fresh fruit and vegetables as snacks. Those changes and others should be coupled with increased, regular physical activity to help children maintain a normal weight over time.

Schools can also play an important role in solving the problem of childhood obesity. Recently, some school districts have come up with interesting strategies. One of these involves engaging more children in physical activities in school that are not organized sports or skill oriented. The state of West Virginia, with one of the highest rates of obesity in the nation, has agreed to install a video game called Dance Dance Revolution (DDR) in all of its 765 public schools in 2008. The game involves moving to a song and shifting directions. Players can dance by themselves or with a partner. The game requires that players process information while doing the various dance moves. For schools and students, the attractions of a game like DDR are many and diverse: It is a new kind of physical education that is noncompetitive, children do not need special equipment or a special place to play it, and it appeals to children who feel they lack the skills and coordination required by organized team sports. Most importantly, it encourages lifetime fitness.

Changing the Environment

Towns and cities in all regions of the nation are finding ways to change the physical environment to get people to become more physically active. Many of their solutions are inexpensive and take a commonsense approach. For example, some towns have built sidewalks and crosswalks in downtown shopping areas to encourage people to walk from store to store. Other solutions such as tearing up derelict railroad tracks and converting the space into walkways and bicycle paths offer health benefits and also beautify the landscape. By holding community-wide health fairs, walking marathons, and fun runs, many town mayors hope to get citizens involved in changing their habits.

In 2007, the city of Somerville, Massachusetts, a suburb of Boston, took a community-wide approach in the battle against obesity. In a controlled experiment devised by researchers at the Tufts School of Nutrition and funded by a grant from the Centers for Disease Control and Prevention (CDC), the children of Somerville were challenged to burn more calories through exercise and take in fewer calories with a healthier diet, for a total benefit of 125 calories a day. The city was made more pedestrian friendly so children could walk to school. School cafeterias altered their menus to include tasty, low-calorie foods that featured fresh fruit, vegetables, and whole grain breads. Student interest in the experiment was prolonged through surveys about the new food offerings. The long-range goal of Somerville's Shape Up plan is to help children graduate from high school at a normal weight.

More Help Is Needed

One of the most vexing problems in the struggle against childhood obesity is the relationship between poverty and obesity. Many poor families equate large servings of high-calorie food as economically advantageous, especially if they are only having one or two meals a day. And many poor neighborhoods lack the kinds of stores that would carry nutritious and fresh foods. Lastly, many obese children live in communities where their parents are reluctant to let them walk to school or to a friend's house or play in a playground or park. Private foundations have taken an interest in helping combat the public health danger of childhood obesity because they regard government funding as inadequate. In 2007, for example, the Robert Wood Johnson Foundation announced a plan to spend more than $500 million over the next five years to reverse the increase in childhood obesity. The money will be used to improve access to healthy food, encourage safe play spaces, and prod governments into adopting policies to address the problem. Reversing the national trend of childhood obesity will not be accomplished in a year or ten years but all agree that it must happen if children are to have long and healthy lives.

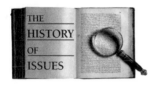

CHAPTER 1

The Origins
of Public Health

Chapter Preface

Public health systems grew out of society's response to combating disease and protecting populations. Because the ancients had no cures for diseases, their only option was to try to explain the causes of illness and take preventive measures to protect health. The ancient Chinese developed an entire system of medicine focused on stimulating the body's own curative powers. Traditional Chinese medicine uses acupuncture, herbal medicine, and exercise and is still practiced today. It is an integral part of China's public health system.

Eventually, humans realized the importance of a clean environment to health. City dwellers in particular saw the need for access to pure drinking water and efficient methods of disposing of the waste they created. In ancient Rome this civic need led to the building of the first public works projects such as aqueducts and sewer systems. In modern times the city of London took a giant step in solving its urban pollution problem by copying and perfecting the sewer system of imperial Rome. Protection of the water supply also figured prominently in the evolution of public health systems.

Society's belief that it had an obligation to care for the well-being of strangers or the less fortunate also led to the development of public health systems. In the early Christian church, for example, religious bodies such as monasteries were required by their rule to provide shelter for travelers, the sick, the elderly, the orphaned, and the insane. Many private philanthropists were inspired by religious ideals to extend charity to the unfortunate by building shelters called hospitals. These institutions were the forerunners of modern public hospitals and mental asylums. By the thirteenth century most towns and cities in Europe operated hospitals for anyone in need.

The appearance of plague in human settlements led to the first organized attempt to control public health. Quarantine, the isolation of the sick person from the rest of the population, was the earliest method of protecting the public's health and with it, the economic life of the community. The plague was easily carried on board ships via infected rats and usually appeared in port cities where it spread into the surrounding countryside. Thus, cities with commercial ties were the first ones to impose rules restricting the movement of anyone suspected of carrying a disease. Their livelihood depended on such laws. In the sixth century A.D. the Byzantine emperor Justinian I ruled that people arriving in the city of Constantinople from regions infected with plague should be hindered in their movements and isolated from the rest of the population. In 1348 the city council of Venice established the world's first organized system of quarantine when it imposed a forty-day waiting period (called a *quaranta giorni*) on any ship desiring to enter its port. Quarantine became government's most utilized method of protecting the public health.

The following chapter traces the development of public works projects such as water and sanitation systems and the impact they had on the public's health. The evolution of laws regarding the protection of public health from earliest times to the founding of the American colonies is also examined.

Public Works Projects in Ancient Rome Provide Sanitation and Clean Water

Roger D. Hansen

The engineers of ancient Rome beautified their city by building arenas, temples, and vast forums. They were also practical men who saw the need for public works projects that would improve the quality of life for Romans. In the following selection, Roger D. Hansen describes the water supply and wastewater systems of ancient Rome and their impact on living conditions in the imperial city.

Like other ancient peoples, the early Romans looked to streams, rainwater catch-basins and especially their river, the Tiber, as sources of water. The Tiber was also used as a place to dispose of sewage. In very little time the river became polluted. It was this environmental disaster that led to the construction of the first aqueduct around 312 B.C. Hansen indirectly makes the point that the aqueducts of ancient Rome led to the rise of a new group of civil servants: the city's water officials. Their vigilance and continual round of repairs kept the water flowing. Despite the abundance of water, the supply to Romans was hardly democratic: The rich and influential could pay to have it piped directly into their homes while the poor had to rely on public fountains.

One of the benefits of living in ancient Rome was the presence of public baths and latrines. Unlike modern on-demand plumbing with its on-and-off controls, water flowed continually into the latrines of ancient Rome and was carried away into a network of sewers. The largest of these was the Cloaca Maxima. And although sewage mixed with rainwater and wastewater, the system was the most advanced in the world at the time.

Roger D. Hansen, "Water and Wastewater Systems in Imperial Rome," *waterhistory.org*, March 8, 2007. Reproduced by permission.

Roger D. Hansen is a historian and civil engineer. He works as a planning team leader in the Office of the Bureau of Reclamation in Provo, Utah.

While much is known about the city's monumental structures like the Coliseum and Forum, less is known about residential structures. Archaeologists tell us that the majority of Romans lived near the center of the city. In an era when urban transportation and communication was slow and difficult, it made sense to concentrate as many residents as possible near centers of attraction. A visitor to ancient Rome generally had trouble getting around. Most of the residential streets were unnamed, and houses and apartments were unnumbered. There were few sidewalks. Streets were narrow and crowded. . . .

Walking Rome's street was frequently dangerous, for it was not unusual to dispose of trash by throwing it out windows.

While there were palaces and individual houses which provided lodging for the rich and powerful, the majority of Romans lived in tenement houses. Because continual rebuilding has destroyed most of Rome's ancient apartments, we need to look at nearby Ostia for information. During the first and second centuries A.D., Ostia was the port of the city of Rome. Silt, along with the decline of the Roman Empire, killed Ostia. The Tiber River delta gradually became unnavigable. The silting up of the Tiber created at Ostia what the cataclismic eruption of Vesuvius created at Pompeii: a wealth of information on domestic life in ancient Rome. . . .

Most of Rome's dwellings were ill-supplied with heat, light, and water. The sanitary arrangements, if judged by modern standards, were inadequate. The typical Roman must have lived almost entirely outside of his tenement house, in the streets, shops, latrines, baths, and arenas of the city. The domicile must have served principally as a place to sleep and store possessions.

The Aqueducts Supply Water to Rome

Romans, at first, turned to the Tiber River, local springs, and shallow wells for their drinking water; but water obtained from these sources grew polluted and became inadequate for the city's growing population. It was this necessity that led to the development of aqueduct technology. The date of the first aqueduct is assigned to the year 312 B.C.

During the time of [Roman engineer and author] Frontinus, nine aqueducts conveyed water from distant springs and streams to Rome. The water in the aqueducts descended gently through concrete channels. Multi-tiered viaducts were used to cross low areas. Inverted siphons were employed (sparingly) when valleys were particularly deep. Tunnels, burrowed through hills too difficult to skirt, were equipped with vertical shafts for inspection and cleaning. Debris cleaned from the tunnels was dumped beside the openings to the vertical shafts. Modern archaeologists have been able to locate long abandoned conduits by finding the piles of debris.

Various vestiges of aqueduct bridges are still in evidence in and around modern Rome. The popular but inaccurate image is that Roman aqueducts were elevated throughout their entire length on lines of arches. Roman engineers were very practical; whenever possible the aqueducts followed a steady downhill course at or below ground level. Inverted siphons, viaducts, and tunnels were used sparingly, when difficult conditions could not be met by any other techniques. The system of aqueducts serving Rome had only 5 percent of its total distance supported by viaducts or bridges.

In the long run, the elevated sections were not an unqualified success. Both archeological and written evidence indicate they required extensive and frequent repairs, which entailed lengthy interruptions in the flow of water. ... [T]he Aqua Claudia, which was under construction for 15 years, was repaired after 10 years of use and 9 years of disuse, repaired again 9 years later and worked on once more just four years later. Evidence of substandard construction and repair work is evident in the sections of the aqueduct that still exist.

To further complicate matters, not all the water diverted into the aqueduct arrived in Rome. Frontinus described the problem of illegal connections:

> ... a large number of landed proprietors, past whose fields the aqueducts run, tap the conduits; whence it comes that the public water courses are actually brought to a standstill by private citizens, just to water their gardens.

Providing Rome an adequate water supply required a constant vigil on the part of water officials.

The aqueduct channels were equipped with air vents or inspection holes. The channels were usually rectangular in the cross-section and varied from 0.5 to 2.0 meters in width and from 1.5 to 2.5 meters in depth. Sometimes two or three channels were superimposed, the upper ones being added to the original to accommodate increasing demand.

Once in or near Rome, water from the aqueducts passed into large, covered catch-basins. Here waters were supposed to deposit their sediment. Waters from the catch-basins were distributed through free-flowing canals, lead pipes, and terra-cotta pipes to storage reservoirs and then through lead pipes (called *fistulae*) to users. The number of connections to private customers were limited; most Romans were obliged to get their supply of domestic water from public fountains.

Water was supposedly only piped into the abodes of those lucky enough to have official authorization, but having running water was so desirable that Romans were constantly bribing water officials to tap an aqueduct. . . .

Getting Clean Water to the City

As one might expect, Roman water quality standards were remedial, taking into consideration only such factors as taste, temperature, smell, and appearance. Since the quality of water from the nine aqueducts varied, the worst waters were used for artificial lakes and irrigation, and the best for drinking. The aqueducts carrying water to Rome were covered to prevent the water from being contaminated by dust, dirt, and other impurities and from being heated by the sun. The best quality waters came from the valley of the Anio River.

One source (Anio Novus) from that watershed, however, did have a water quality problem every time it rained. Roman engineers first tried mixing it with water from a nearby clear spring. Next they tried running it through a small settling basin. Because of design problems with the basin, this too was unsuccessful. Finally the condition of the water was improved by carrying the head of the aqueduct higher up the valley to a reservoir formed behind an immense dam near Subiaco. The artificial lake served efficiently as a settling basin and the quality of the water was improved.

The dam at Subiaco was built to form a pleasure lake for the Emperor Nero. It was a straight masonry dam and reached a maximum height of approximately 40 meters. The Subiaco Dam was the highest such structure built by the Romans and their only known use of dam technology in Italy. It failed in A.D. 1305 without leaving a trace.

It has been hypothesized that Rome's dependence on lead water pipes led to its decline. It has been suggested that the aristocracy died off from nothing more complicated than simple lead poisoning.

Since almost all of the lead absorbed by the human body is deposited in bones, investigators have studied the bones of ancient Romans. While some studies did indicate above normal concentrations of lead, it seems unlikely that water pipes were a contributing factor . . . for two reasons: (1) because the Roman water contained high concentrations of calcium which formed deposits inside the pipes, insulating the lead and (2) because lead will never greatly affect running water.

Water to the Houses, Latrines, and Baths

Water was provided for a variety of uses including fountains (which served as sources for culinary water) and latrines, and for more exotic activities such as public baths and sham naval battles. With few exceptions, the water from the aqueducts reached only the ground floor of apartment buildings. The tenants of the upper floors had to rely on slaves to carry water or go themselves and draw water from the nearest fountain. Because fire was a constant concern, Romans were encouraged to keep water stored in their rooms.

It is not difficult to imagine the problem sixth-floor residents, with no running water, had in dealing with fire and public sanitation. Residents of apartment buildings lived with a constant fear of fire. . . .

Many must also have lived in a constant state of squalor. In fact, fire probably served an important public sanitation function.

We know that Rome was struck by massive fires on several occasions. Most notable was the fire during the reign of the Emperor Nero which destroyed large sections of Rome because the city had no effective means of stopping the spread of the fire. . . .

Besides private connections and fountains, the aqueducts supplied water to latrines. Many of Rome's were sumptuous. All around the circular or rectangular structure, water flowed continuously in small channels. One of the more elaborate establishments had 20 seats made of marble and each seat was framed by sculptured brackets in the form of dolphins. Occasionally the latrine was cheered by the sounds and sights of a fountain. Latrines were heated; nothing is colder than marble.

Two common forms of entertainment—baths and sham naval battles required large quantifies of water. During the Roman Empire, baths became more and more elaborate, providing not only bathing facilities, but games, lectures, musical performances, prostitutes, calisthenics, and places to lounge and gossip. The baths had hot, warm, and cold water pools. The water in the pools was changed several times each day. The air and water were heated by a number of underground furnaces. These furnaces were like bakers' ovens. Water of two different temperatures—hot and warm—circulated automatically by thermo-siphon. . . .

How Much Water and for How Many?

One unresolved historical problem regarding water use bears discussion; the quantity of water provided by the aqueducts. In general, data provided by archeological evidence and written accounts fall short of that required for the computation of either per capita supply or per capita use. The cross-sectional areas of the aqueducts are known, but one cannot be sure the conduits ever ran full. Sizing of the channels was probably determined as much by the need for work space as by the volume needed for water. As previously mentioned, it was certainly a rare occasion when the aqueducts were all working at the same time. Another uncertainty is the population of Imperial Rome. No accurate estimate exists for any particular period. It is generally assumed that during Frontinus' era the population of Rome was approximately one million.

Early opinions on the amount of water delivered by the aqueducts varies from a low of 322,000 cubic meters per day to a high of 1,010,623. There is also little consensus among more recent estimates. . . .

The Romans also diverted water into storage tanks. Archaeologists have uncovered large cisterns in Rome, many received water from the aqueducts. . . .

It is safe to assume that Rome received an impressive supply of water, and that the rich and influential received a disproportionate amount. But the water supply for the common Roman was still sufficient. By historic standards, Rome's water supply was a very impressive accomplishment.

Drains and Sewers Were
Well Constructed but Underused

Water from the baths, latrines, palaces, fountains, etc., as well as other urban runoff was discharged into Rome's drainage and wastewater collection system. Several centuries before the birth of Christ, Etruscan engineers built the initial drainage system (Cloaca Maxima) whose main outlet into the Tiber River still exists 28 centuries later. The covered drains were designed on such a large scale that in certain sections wagons loaded with hay could drive through with ease. Rome's sewers and drains emptied directly into the Tiber, whose polluted state must have been a constant problem for the Roman populace.

The Roman sewers have been overpraised. Despite their longevity, they ignored basic sanitary principles. They carried sewage, urban runoff, and drainage water together. This multiple employment made it necessary to have large openings along the streets. These openings exposed Rome's populace to the effluvia of the sewers. To mitigate this danger to public health, Romans had only two protections: (1) the masses of water from infiltration and the aqueducts which constantly flushed the drains, and (2) the hilly nature of the city which gave the drains a steep slope.

The Roman sewer system probably carried off at least as much water as the aqueducts provided. Consumptive use in Rome was not high and there was a lot of infiltration into the drains from groundwater (parts of Rome are constructed over swamps). The flow of the Tiber River was greatly increased by discharges from Rome's sewers.

Although the ancient sewers were very skillfully constructed, they were not used to their full potential. There were few private connections to the sewers. Even with the wastewater system's shortcoming, it is astonishing to note the absence of significant improvements in collection systems until the 1840's, some 17 centuries later.

Monasteries, Hospitals, and Hospices Were the Public Health System in Medieval Europe

James William Brodman

In western Europe during the medieval period, monasteries run by religious orders such as the Benedictines were obligated by the rules of their order to take in the poor and needy. In addition, towns and cities took measures to provide food and shelter for the poor, the homeless, and travelers. Their motivations sprang from a sense of charity but also from practical concerns such as ensuring safety and the public order. A concept of government oversight for public health gradually evolved from this setting.

Author James W. Brodman examines the role of hospitals in medieval Spain in the following selection. In addition to the work performed by monasteries and other communities on behalf of the needy, cities from Spain to England built shelters (called hospitals) that provided housing and food for the traveler, the religious pilgrim, the homeless, the aged poor, and the chronically infirm. They also took in the sick and those suffering from dreaded diseases such as leprosy. The institutions remained semireligious in nature but were governed by boards of directors and endowed by the community, private individuals, or local nobility. By the 1300s these institutions became more concerned with aiding the sick than with providing shelter. Thus, they became the model for the modern public hospital.

James W. Brodman is the director of the Library of Iberian Resources Online of the Department of History, University of Central Arkansas.

Shelter for the temporarily homeless, whether or not they were needy in the modern sense, was as typical a charity in the towns and villages of medieval Europe as was providing food to the hungry. The Rule of Saint Benedict, as well as local Hispanic customs, imposed the obligation of hospitality upon monasteries. Likewise, in the reviving towns of the eleventh and twelfth centuries, there was a need to provide beds for those who were not householders. Urban hospices served a diverse lot: pilgrims wending their way to a shrine like Santiago, clergy and others in town on business, wandering beggars, and the local poor. Increasingly, those with means seem to have secured their own accommodation in inns or residences, while paupers sought out the more public shelters operated by churches, monasteries, town government, and even private individuals. By the thirteenth century, every town of size in Europe, including Iberia, had several of these shelters. The texts describe these institutions as hospitals or, less frequently, by the old Byzantine term *xenodochium*. While they functioned primarily as shelters, these hospitals would at times offer other forms of care because their guests needed refreshment and might also require medical assistance.

The Growth of Cities and the Pilgrim Road Give Rise to Hospitals

The earliest known hospital in Christian Iberia was the *xenodochium* established by Bishop Masona at Mérida in 580, but, in post-Visigothic times, the stimulus of urban development and the pilgrim road to Santiago gave rise to many hospitals in the northern portion of the peninsula. This was a new development of the eleventh and twelfth centuries. Studies at León, for example, have demonstrated that older benefactions to its cathedral would form no part of the endowments of the . . . shelters that began to appear just before 1100. These shelters served the local poor and sick, but especially pilgrims who were often in as much need of care as shelter, given the dangers of the journey and the preexisting illnesses that motivated many pilgrimages. Thus, in 1052 King García Sánchez III of Navarre established the hospice of Santa María de Nájera; at León, in 1084 Bishop Pelayo opened a place near the cathedral for the sick, lame, blind, deaf, and hungry, as well as for pilgrims, and, twelve years later, Bishop Pedro moved it to a larger site just outside of town; Archbishop Gelmírez of Santiago in the early twelfth century followed this precedent. Elsewhere along this pilgrim route, we find the Hospital de San Juan in Oviedo, where the feet of pilgrims were washed, the late tenth-century Hospital de la Trinidad de Arre, near Pamplona, the eleventh-century Hospital de San Esteban at Astorga, the Hospital de Santa Cristina at the pass of Somport, and the early twelfth-century hospices at Aubrac and Roncesvalles in the Pyrenees. In Burgos, among some thirty known hospitals, were the Hospital del Rey, the Hospital del Emperador, and the Hospital de Santa María la Real, all of which specialized in sheltering pilgrims on the Santiago road, the Hospital de San Lucas that housed invalids, and a ... hospice near the cathedral for the local paupers. Other, smaller institutions served the needs of specific parishes ... Elsewhere, Astorga had twenty hospitals and Salamanca twenty-eight. León's first hospital was the episcopal Hospital de San Juan (1084), and by 1250 it was joined by eight others. At Valladolid, the Hospital de Esgueva, which dated from the end of the eleventh century, was but one of twenty institutions in the fifteenth century. Seville, a Castilian town only after 1248, had five hospitals by 1300 that included pilgrim hospices established by King Alfonso X and another by Aragonese settlers in the region; five others were founded in the fourteenth century, including that of San Bernando for poor, elderly residents of the town. Córdoba counted at least thirty-three hospital establishments founded in the thirteenth and fourteenth centuries. Valencia, another "new" city, saw a half dozen hospitals established in the immediate decades after its conquest, most under ecclesiastical governance, and by the fifteenth century this number had risen to fourteen. Thirteenth-century Saragossa had eleven hospitals and Toulouse more than a dozen. In Portugal, there were over forty-seven hospices just north of the Douro, and another twenty-five leprosaria [hospitals for lepers]; the town of Porto itself had eight hospitals.

The Iberian phenomenon was typical of the situation elsewhere in Europe. In Paris, there was the large Hôtel-Dieu near Notre Dame Cathedral for transients and the sick, as well as other hospices for lepers, pilgrims, orphans, ex-prostitutes, and the blind. Paris itself had about sixty hospitals in all, and the smaller towns of Narbonne, and Arles had fifteen and sixteen. The chronicler Giovanni Villani reports that Florence had about thirty hospitals at the beginning of the fourteenth century, and a century later there were ten more. In 1350 Rome counted twenty-five. In the Low Countries, there is record of pilgrim hospices from 1137 and of urban hospitals from 1090 (at Louvain). In 1154, England had 113 known hospitals, and more than 700 by 1300, not counting monastic infirmaries, establishments of the Hospitallers of Saint John and the ubiquitous small, undocumented establishments. Thus, the phenomenon of public shelters was one that Catalonia shared with the rest of Europe.

Many Providers, Many Shelters

While the oldest hospital in Catalonia will likely never be identified, two of the earliest were the hospices for pilgrims and travelers located at the Benedictine monasteries of Sant Pere de Rodes, which dates from the late tenth century, and of Sant Pere de Casserres, which was founded in the eleventh century. Both were constructed outside the monastic walls as simple two-storied hostels. At around the same time, the count of Cerdanya in 965 established a hospice for travelers at the Coll de la Perxa, a deserted spot on the road from Cerdanya to the Conflent, which was served by a community of lay brothers and servants. There were other refuges at the Hills of Puymorens and Arnés, and at Sentillà and Santa Cecília de Rella. In the valley of Clusa three other hospices for pilgrims depended on the monasteries of Sant Hilarde Rasez, Arlés and Soreda. Instances of other such shelters, located in towns, villages, and rural locales, proliferate during the eleventh century. At Barcelona, Bishop Deodat donated to a hospital for the poor in 1024, and another named "En Guitard" was established circa 1045, the same year someone named Arnau opened a hospital for the poor next to the cathedral at Urgell; Girona possibly had a hospital within the old Roman fortifications in the tenth century. Another hospital was established at Cardona in 1083, and in 1068 Arsendis, the wife of Arnau Mir of Tost, asked her spouse to establish shelters for the infirm poor at Tost as well as at Algar, Montmagastre, and Artesa. In the eleventh century Vic had an *Albergueria*, located behind the cathedral, that served as a residence for clergy as well as a hospital. At the beginning of the next century, in 1101, the chapter of Ager established a shelter for travelers, and, in 1116, Count Arnau de Roselló instituted a shelter for Christ's poor at the Church of Sant Joan at Perpignan.

Throughout Catalonia, as indeed throughout Christian Iberia and western Europe, bishops, chapters, confraternities, prosperous and perhaps pious individuals, and eventually even municipalities established a myriad of such shelters to house and, at times, offer various types of material assistance to an assortment of temporarily or permanently homeless persons: travelers and pilgrims, the old, the sick and the dying, and the destitute. . . .

Public shelters were not confined to the Christian community. . . . In 1277, Abraham of Alexandria and his son, Astruc, the founder of the *almoina* for the Jewish community of Barcelona, endowed a hospice for the poor and travelers in a house of the call (or Jewish quarter) that had been established earlier by Rabbi Samuel ben rabí Isaac Ha-Sardí, a native of Cerdanya. At the end of the fourteenth century, it was known as the hospital of the poor Jews, and was governed by four hospitallers or proctors. A document of 1385 records the gift of a bed made from four boards, a mattress, a bolster, and associated bedding. Despite such gifts, however, this and other charities in Jewish *aljamas* [temples] were actually funded by an informal system of taxation, in which each man was expected to pay stated assessments and also make voluntary contributions. The destruction of the Jewish quarter in the riots of 1391, however, probably eliminated the hospital. . . .

A Narrower View of Hospitals Emerges Around the 1300s

If the idea of the public shelter, whose purpose was to assist anyone who needed lodging, germinated shortly after the year 1000, it came to bloom and flourished in the twelfth and thirteenth centuries when towns, large and small, and rural locales as well, supported one or more of these establishments. The initiative for their creation was for the most part episcopal, but by the twelfth century wealthy individuals, clerical and lay, and religious communities also served as sponsors and patrons. A century later, municipal governments began to assume some responsibility for sheltering the poor. Those establishments in rural locales and in the smaller towns tended to retain more of their initial character as shelters for travelers and pilgrims, as well as the local poor. Urban hospices, on the other hand, seemed to have paid as much attention to needy residents as to transients. By the fourteenth century, the idea that the primary purpose of a hospital was the provision of bed and board would be on the wane, with the appearance of new institutions who saw their function in narrower terms, to treat disease and other physical ills. The earlier concept of serving all of the poor, however, was not entirely lost. This evolution of function can be seen in the admission policies of

Valencia's Hospital of En Clapers. Founded by a merchant in 1311, it served various classes of the sick but refused entry to those whose disability was merely material. Nonetheless, the poor were not entirely ignored by En Clapers, because small alms, handfuls of pennies, were dispensed to those who came begging for food. As for travelers with means, however, the provision of shelter increasingly became a commercial enterprise, as private homes, hostels, and taverns began to take in paying guests.

Plague Forces Cities to Develop Laws to Protect the Public Health

Marchione di Coppo Stefani (Part I) and
Simone Buonacorsi (Part II)

The year 1348 marked a momentous event in the history of western European civilization: the arrival of the bubonic plague. The plague spread through the countryside of Europe and devastated the cities and towns where it struck. Historians estimate that up to two-thirds of the population of many large European cities perished as a result of the plague in the first two years. Many people of the time explained the plague as a curse of God or as an infestation brought about by women, lepers, or Jews. More rational minds saw it as a disease that defied treatment. Leaders of cities and regions took measures such as quarantine and limiting travel to protect the populace from the disease but to little avail. Additionally, they organized efficient ways to deal with the dead. As a result of the responses of local governments, the plague did much to heighten Europeans' understanding of public health.

The plague and how governments reacted to it is the subject of the following two selections. The first selection is taken from The Florentine Chronicle *by Marchione di Coppo Stefani and gives a detailed account of the plague's effect on the city of Florence. The second selection is from the "Ordinances for Sanitation in a Time of Mortality" issued by the governing council of the city of Pistoia. Both selections reveal the medical and ethical issues facing city leaders when faced with a rampaging disease.*

Part I: Marchione di Coppo Stefani, "Rubric 643: Concerning A Mortality In The City Of Florence In Which Many People Died," *The Florentine Chronicle*, 1370-1380. Part II: Simone Buonacorsi, from *Ordinances for Sanitation in a Time of Mortality*, 1348.

Part I: Plague in Florence

In the year of the Lord 1348 there was a very great pestilence in the city and district of Florence. It was of such a fury and so tempestuous that in houses in which it took hold previously healthy servants who took care of the ill died of the same illness. Almost non[e] of the ill survived past the fourth day. Neither physicians nor medicines were effective. Whether because these illnesses were previously unknown or because physicians had not previously studied them, there seemed to be no cure. There was such a fear that no one seemed to know what to do. When it took hold in a house it often happened that no one remained who had not died. And it was not just that men and women died, but even sentient animals died. Dogs, cats, chickens, oxen, donkeys, sheep showed the same symptoms and died of the same disease. And almost none, or very few, who showed these symptoms, were cured. The symptoms were the following: a bubo [swelling] in the groin, where the thigh meets the trunk; or a small swelling under the armpit; sudden fever; spitting blood and saliva (and no one who spit blood survived it). It was such a frightful thing that when it got into a house, as was said, no one remained. Frightened people abandoned the house and fled to another. Those in town fled to villages. Physicians could not be found because they had died like the others. And those who could be found wanted vast sums in hand before they entered the house. And when they did enter, they checked the pulse with face turned away. They inspected the urine from a distance and with something odoriferous under their nose. Child abandoned the father, husband the wife, wife the husband, one brother the other, one sister the other. In all the city there was nothing to do but to carry the dead to a burial. And those who died had neither confessor nor other sacraments. And many died with no one looking after them. And many died of hunger because when someone took to bed sick, another in the house, terrified, said to him: "I'm going for the doctor." Calmly walking out the door, the other left and did not return again. . . .

Dealing with the Dead

Many died unseen. So they remained in their beds until they stank. And the neighbors, if there were any, having smelled the stench, placed them in a shroud and sent them for burial. The house remained open and yet there was no one daring enough to touch anything because it seemed that things remained poisoned and that whoever used them picked up the illness.

At every church, or at most of them, they dug deep trenches, down to the waterline, wide and deep, depending on how large the parish was. And those who were responsible for the dead carried them on their backs in the night in which they died and threw them into the ditch, or else they paid a high price to those who would do it for them. The next morning, if there were many [bodies] in the trench, they covered them over with dirt. And then more bodies were put on top of them, with a little more dirt over those; they put layer on layer just like one puts layers of cheese in a lasagna.

The beccamorti [literally vultures] who provided their service, were paid such a high price that many were enriched by it. Many died from [carrying away the dead] some rich, some after earning just a little, but high prices continued. Servants, or those who took care of the ill, charged from one to three florins per day and the cost of things grew. The things that the sick ate, sweetmeats and sugar, seemed priceless. Sugar cost from three to eight florins per pound. And other confections cost similarly. Capons and other poultry were very expensive and eggs cost between twelve and twenty-four pence each; and he was blessed who could find three per day even if he searched the entire city. Finding wax was miraculous. A pound of wax would have gone up more than a florin if there had not been a stop put [by the communal government] to the vain ostentation that the Florentines always make [over funerals]. Thus it was ordered that no more than two large candles could be carried [in any funeral]. Churches had no more than a single bier which usually was not sufficient. Spice dealers and beccamorti sold biers, burial palls, and cushions at very high prices. Dressing in expensive woolen cloth as is customary in [mourning] the dead, that is in a long cloak, with mantle and veil that used to cost women three florins climbed in price to thirty florins and would have climbed to 100 florins had the custom of dressing in expensive cloth not been changed. The rich dressed in modest woolens, those not rich sewed [clothes] in linen. Benches on which the dead were placed cost like the heavens and still the benches were only a hundredth of those needed. Priests were not able to ring bells as they would have liked. Concerning that [the government] issued ordinances discouraging the sounding of bells, sale of burial benches, and limiting expenses. They could not sound bells, sell benches, nor cry out announcements because the sick hated to hear of this and it discouraged the healthy as well. Priests and friars went [to serve] the rich in great multitudes and they were paid such high prices that they all got rich. And therefore [the authorities] ordered that one could not have more than a prescribed number [of clerics] of the local parish church. And the prescribed number of friars was six. All fruits with a nut at the center, like unripe plums and unhusked almonds, fresh broadbeans, figs and every useless and unhealthy fruit, were forbidden entrance into the city. Many processions, including those with relics and the painted tablet of Santa Maria Inpruneta, went through the city crying our "Mercy" and praying and then they came to a stop in the piazza of the Priors. There they made peace concerning important controversies, injuries and deaths.

Impact on the City

This [pestilence] was a matter of such great discouragement and fear that men gathered together in order to take some comfort in dining together. And each evening one of them provided dinner to ten companions and the next evening they planned to eat with one of the others. And sometimes if they planned to eat with a certain one he had no meal prepared because he was sick. Or if the host had made dinner for the ten, two or three were missing. Some fled to villas, others to villages in order to get a change of air. Where there had been no [pestilence], there they carried it; if it was already there, they caused it to increase. None of the guilds in Florence was working. All the shops were shut, taverns closed; only the apothecaries and the churches remained open. If you went outside, you found almost no one. And many good and rich men were carried from home to church on a pall by four beccamorti and one tonsured clerk who carried the cross. Each of them wanted a florin. . . .

This pestilence began in March, as was said, and ended in September 1348. And people began to return to look after their houses and possessions. And there were so many houses full of goods without a master that it was stupefying. Then those who would inherit these goods began to appear. And such it was that those who had nothing found themselves rich with what did not seem to be theirs and they were unseemly because of it. Women and men began to dress ostentatiously.

Part II: Laws of Pistoia Concerning the Plague

In the name of Christ, Amen. Herein are written certain ordinances and provisions made and agreed upon by certain wise men of the People of the city of Pistoia elected and commissioned by the lords Anziani and the Standardbearer of Justice of the said city concerning the preserving, strengthening and protecting the health of humans from various and diverse pestilences which otherwise can befall the human body. And written by me Simone Buonacorsi notary . . . in the year from the Nativity of the Lord MCCCXLVIII, the first Indiction.

First. So that no contaminated matter which presently persists in the areas surrounding the city of Pistoia can enter into the bodies of the citizens of Pistoia, these wise men provided and ordered that no citizen of Pistoia or dweller in the district or the county of Pistoia . . . shall in any way dare or presume to go to Pisa or Lucca or to the county or district of either. And that no one can or ought to come from either of them or their districts . . . to the said city of Pistoia or its district or county on penalty of # [lire] 50. . . . And that gatekeeper of the city of Pistoia guarding the gates of the said city shall not permit those coming or returning to the said city of Pistoia from the said cities of Pisa or Lucca, their districts or counties to enter the said gates on penalty of # 10. . . . It is licit, however, for citizens now living in Pistoia to go to Pisa and Lucca, their districts and counties and then return if they have first obtained a license from the Council of the People. . . .

II. Item. The foresaid wise men provided and ordered that no person whether citizen, inhabitant of the district or county of the city of Pistoia or foreigner shall dare or presume in any way to bring . . . to the city of Pistoia, its district or county, any used cloth, either linen or woolen, for use as clothing for men or women or for bedclothes on penalty of # 200. . . . Citizens of Pistoia, its district and county returning to the city, district or county will be allowed to bring with them the linen or woolen cloths they are wearing and those for personal use carried in luggage or a small bundle weighing 30 pounds or less. . . . And if any quantity of cloth of the said type or quality has been carried into the said city, county or district, the carrier shall be held to and must remove and export it from the said city, county and district within three days of the adoption of the present ordinance under the foresaid penalty for each carrier or carriers and for each violation.

III. Item. They provided and ordered that the bodies of the dead, after they had died, can not be nor ought to be removed from the place in which they are found unless first such a body has been placed in a wooden casket covered by a lid secured with nails, so that no stench can issue forth from it; nor can it be covered except by a canopy, blanket or drape under a penalty for # 50 of pennies paid by the heirs of the dead person. . . . And also that likewise such dead bodies of the dead must be carried to the grave only in the said casket under the said penalty as has been said. And so that the foresaid shall be noted by the rectors and officials of the city of Pistoia, present and future rectors of the parishes of the city of Pistoia in whose parish there is any dead person are held to and must themselves announce the death and the district [of the city] in which the dead person lived to the podesta [chief magistrate] and captain or others of the government of the said city. And they must notify them of the name of the dead person and of the district in which the dead person had lived or pay the said penalty for each contravention. And the podesta and captain to whom such an announcement or notification has been made, immediately are held to and must send one of their officials to the same location to see and inquire if the contents of the present article and other statutes and ordinances concerning funerals are being observed and to punish anyone found culpable according to the said penalty. . . . And the foresaid shall not be enforced nor is it extended to poor and miserable persons who are declared to be poor and miserable according to the form of any statutes or ordinances of the said city.

IV. Item. In order to avoid the foul stench which the bodies of the dead give off they have provided and ordered that any ditch in which a dead body is to be buried must be dug under ground to a depth of 2 1/2 braccia [a unit of measure] by the measure of the city of Pistoia.

V. Item. They have provided and ordered that no person of whatever condition or status or authority shall dare or presume to return or to carry to the city of Pistoia any dead body in or out of a casket or in any manner on penalty of #

25 of pennies paid by whoever carries, brings, or orders [a body] to be carried or brought for each occasion. And that the gatekeepers of the said city shall not permit such a body to be sent into the said city on penalty of the foresaid fine by each gatekeeper at the gate through which the said body was sent.

VI. Item. They have provided and ordered that any person who will have come for the burial or to bury any dead person can not and may not be in the presence of the body itself nor with the relatives of such a dead person except for the procession to the church where it will be buried. Nor shall such persons return to the house where the defunct person lived or enter into that house or any other house on the said occasion on penalty of # 10.

VII. Item. They have provided and ordered that when anyone has died no person should dare or presume to present or to send any gift before or after burial to the former dwelling place of such a dead person or any other place on the said occasion or to attend or to go to a meal in that house or place on the said occasion on penalty of # 25. . . . Children, carnal brothers and sisters, nieces and nephews of such a dead person and their children, however, shall be expected [from this provision].

VIII. Item. They have provided and ordered that in order to avoid useless or fruitless expenses no person should dare or presume to dress in new clothing during the period of mourning for any dead person or during the eight days after that, on penalty of # 25 of pennies for whoever contravenes [this] and for each time. Wives of such dead persons, however, shall be exempted; they can be dressed in whatever new clothing they wish without penalty.

IX. Item. They have provided and ordered that no paid mourner . . . shall dare or presume to mourn publicly or privately or to invite other citizens of Pistoia to go to the funeral or to the dead person; nor may anyone engage the foresaid mourner, hornplayer, cryer or drummer.

X. Item. So that the sounds of bells might not depress the infirm nor fear arise in them [the Wise Men] have provided and ordered that the bellringers or custodians in charge of the belltower of the cathedral of Pistoia shall not permit any bell in the said campanile [bell tower] to be rung for the funeral of the dead nor shall any person dare or presume to ring any of these bells on the said occasion. . . .

XIV. Item. They have provided and ordered that butchers and retail vendors of meat, individually and in common, can not, nor ought to hold or maintain near a tavern or other place where they sell meats, or near a shop or beside or behind a shop any stable, pen or any other thing which will give off a putrid smell; nor can they slaughter meat animals nor hang them after slaughter in any stable or other place in which there is any stench on a penalty of # 10.

XXII. Item. So that stench and putrefaction shall not be harmful to men, henceforth tanning of hides can not and must not be done within the walls of the city of Pistoia on penalty of # 25. . . .

XXIII. Item. For the observance of each and every provision contained in the present articles and everything in the article speaking of funerals of the dead, of butchers and retail vendors of meats, . . . officials charged pro tem with the foresaid [duties] shall and must proceed against, investigate, and inquire . . . concerning acts contrary to the foresaid [ordinances], and cause whatever of the foresaid ordained to be reviewed as often as possible, and punish the guilty by the foresaid fines. . . .

London Builds a Huge Sewer System to Cleanse the Crowded City

National Maritime Museum

By the middle of the nineteenth century London was one of the most populated and most polluted cities in the world. The city's teeming populace used the river Thames as their sewer and also as a main source of drinking water. Industries dumped their toxic wastes into the Thames, further exacerbating the pollution. Londoners were stricken by several cholera epidemics in the 1800s as a consequence of their polluted water and fouled environment. Bad smells from the river were particularly offensive. London had become a dangerously noxious place.

By 1858, the city government was ready to tackle the problem of waste disposal. The circumstances surrounding the development of London's sewer system is the topic of the following selection. The sewer system, still in existence today, was the work of Joseph Bazalgette, the chief engineer of the Metropolitan Board of Works. Bazalgette's scheme involved gathering sewage and moving it east of London. Over the years the system evolved from dumping waste to treating it with chemicals, and then dumping the sludge at sea. Today, sludge is no longer dumped at sea and is incinerated instead. Bazalgette's accomplishment proved the importance of public works to improve the environment and protect the public health.

By the middle of the 19th century, London was on the brink of an environmental catastrophe. The city was growing rapidly in terms of population and size, and the old ways of supplying water, burying the dead and disposing of sewage were rapidly becoming inadequate.

National Maritime Museum, "Bazalgette and London's Sewage," *portcities.org.uk*, March 23, 2007. Reproduced by permission.

Little was done until the 'Great Stink' of 1858 offended Members of Parliament. Over the following seven years, Joseph Bazalgette and the Metropolitan Board of Works constructed a simple but immense sewage disposal system for London, an awesome feat for the time. London still relies on Bazalgette's sewers.

The Thames Becomes a Sewer

For centuries, human waste had been removed from the cesspits as 'night soil' and taken away for use as fertilizer on fields around London.

With the relentless growth of London, this was no longer feasible. The population of London doubled between 1801 and 1841, and the city was rapidly spreading outwards. Most houses used cesspits, which often overflowed through the floorboards. Many cesspits emptied into open sewers or the tributaries of the Thames.

With the situation worsening, something was finally done in 1847. The Metropolitan Commission of Sewers was formed to tackle the problem.

The Commission's first act was to close the cesspits. This turned out to be a disaster, as the city's sewage now found its way into the Thames.

Before long, the river itself was little more than a sewer. Londoners were quick to notice how rapidly their river had declined. The satirical magazine *Punch* published several memorable cartoons deploring the disgusting state of the Thames.

The smell was only a small part of the problem, as London obtained most of its drinking water from the Thames. This made Londoners particularly vulnerable to water-borne diseases such as cholera.

The first cholera pandemic began in India in 1817 and spread outwards to Europe, reaching Britain in 1831–32. In just over a year, around 31,000 died from the disease. London's first case occurred in February 1832, and at least 6,000 died in the capital. Later outbreaks killed 54,000 people in Britain in 1848–49 (including 14,000 in London) and 31,000 in 1853–54 (10,000 in London).

During the third epidemic, Dr John Snow proved that cholera was a water-borne disease, but few medical men believed him at the time. Most still supported the miasma theory, which stated that disease was caused by foul air from rotting matter and stagnant water.

Bad Smells

In 1856 the Metropolitan Board of Works had been formed to carry out large public works in London, including the construction of a sewage disposal system. However, it did not have sufficient funds for such a task.

As so often before—and since—very little was done until powerful people felt their interests were being threatened.

For many years, the smell caused by sewage in the Thames became particularly unbearable during the summer.

During the summer of 1858 it was so bad that even Members of Parliament suffered, and curtains soaked in chemicals were used to keep the smell out of the House of Commons. Unsurprisingly, the necessary funds for a sewage disposal system were soon made available.

Moving the Sewage Downstream

Once the enabling act was passed, the Metropolitan Board of Works could begin the task under the direction of its Chief Engineer, Joseph Bazalgette (1819–91).

Most schemes for removing London's sewage had planned to carry it inland so it could still be used as fertilizer, but Bazalgette realised this was impractical. Instead, he planned to build main sewers to collect the contents of the existing sewers and take their contents east to be discharged into the Thames.

Bazalgette's scheme consisted of three major elements:

- the intercepting sewers

- the pumping stations and the outfall sewers

- the pumping stations at Beckton and Crossness.

Each of these involved major feats of engineering.

On either side of the Thames, three main intercepting sewers captured the sewage from all existing sewers and carried them by gravity eastwards to the pumping stations at Abbey Mills (for the north bank) and Deptford (for the south).

The pumping stations raised the sewage so it could be carried by gravity to the Thames. It flowed to the river in the massive pipes of the outfall sewers.

The outfall sewers were a massive feat of engineering. The Northern Outfall Sewer was more than 6.5 km (4 miles) long, and crossed the marshes east of the River Lea.

For most of its length, the Northern Outfall Sewer was concealed within a massive embankment. Several bridges carried it across the River Lea and its branches. The scale of the work is still impressive today.

The Southern Outfall Sewer ran underground for much of its length from Deptford to Crossness. At Beckton and Crossness, the sewage was stored in huge reservoirs, from which it was released into the Thames at high tide.

The Embankments on either side of the Thames were another benefit of Bazalgette's scheme. The idea of building embankments to reclaim marshy land along the riverbank had been debated for centuries, but little was done before Bazalgette.

His embankments concealed sections of his intercepting sewers, and avoided the huge cost and inconvenience of digging up central London streets. They reclaimed nearly 10 hectares (22 acres) of mud, and also concealed a section of the Metropolitan Railway, the world's first underground railway line.

The whole scheme took seven years to complete. Bazalgette's achievement was amazing even by modern standards. When completed in 1865, London had 2100 km (1300 miles) of sewers, including 130 km (82 miles) of the main intercepting sewers. Almost a century and a half later, London still relies on Bazalgette's sewers.

Problems Remain

Although Bazalgette's achievement was huge, his system simply shifted the problem downriver. As the sewage was discharged into the Thames untreated, problems were building up. Large mudbanks of sewage began to form downriver from the outfalls. Even worse, the sewage took a long time to clear the Thames, as incoming tides brought it back part of the way.

The dreadful state of the river near the outfalls was highlighted by the *Princess Alice* tragedy of September 1878. The pleasure steamer sank after a collision with a collier in Galleons Reach, not far from Beckton.

Almost cut in half by the force of the impact, the *Princess Alice* sank in less than five minutes. The unfortunate passengers were thrown into the filthiest and most polluted stretch of the river.

Around 650 people died that evening in the biggest ever disaster on the Thames. Few of the victims died in the actual collision—most drowned in the toxic combination of raw sewage and industrial pollutants.

A Royal Commission gathered in 1882 to debate the next step. It recommended chemical treatment of the sewage. From 1887, the liquid effluent was separated from the solid sludge. Only the former was discharged into the river. The sludge was removed by special boats for disposal at sea.

From 1887 to 1898, a fleet of sludge boats made regular journeys from Beckton and Crossness to Barrow Deep beyond the mouth of the Thames. Between 1915 and 1967, the nearby Black Deep site was also used for dumping sludge.

Surprisingly, the best description of the work of London's sludge boats comes from a sermon by the distinguished Methodist preacher William Sangster (1900–60). Always eager to use unconventional associations in his sermons, he used sludge disposal as a metaphor for divine forgiveness.

> London has four sludge vessels. They are tankers really, with a cargo-carrying capacity of 1,500 tons. On every weekday tide, two of the sludge vessels set out laden with this unwanted and perilous matter and travel down the Thames to Black Deep, a depression on the bed of the ocean, fifteen miles off Foulness.

> When the vessel reaches Black Deep, the valves are opened and the complete cargo runs out in about twenty minutes. Down it goes, down into the salt aseptic sea. A dark stain spreads over the wake of the ship, but so wide is the ocean, and so deep the delivery, and so briny the sea that, within one hour, samples of water taken either from the surface of the sea, or the bed of the estuary prove to be completely innocuous. The sludge has gone, devitalized of all evil power, and never to be seen again. . . .

More Changes

Since the 1990s, the treatment of London's sewage has changed again. To comply with European Union legislation forbidding the dumping of sewage at sea, this method has been discontinued.

Around half of London's waste is now incinerated at Crossness and Beckton. The electricity generated from the incineration is sufficient to power the treatment plants, and Beckton even has a surplus to sell back to one National Grid.

Hamburg Struggles
to Deal with Cholera

Annesley Kenealy

Cholera is a contagious disease that spreads by means of water or food tainted by untreated sewage. In the 1800s outbreaks of cholera resulted in the deaths of hundreds of thousands in London, Paris, Saint Petersburg, Russia, and elsewhere. It was not until the discovery of the microorganisms that spread the disease and the rise of the science of bacteriology in the late 1800s and early 1900s that cholera was brought under control. Today, water filtration and chlorination have practically eliminated cholera from the developed world. It still persists, however, in poor, underdeveloped countries.

In the following selection, Annesley Kenealy describes an outbreak of cholera in the German city of Hamburg that resulted in the deaths of over 8 thousand people. Kenealy volunteered to help the sick of that city and her report, delivered to the Women's Congress of the Columbian World Exposition in 1893, is that of an eyewitness. She provides information about how cholera arrived in Hamburg and notes the reactions of the authorities and the medical establishment. Kenealy also comments on the vital role of clean drinking water in preventing the disease. Annesley Kenealy was a native of Sussex, England, and studied at the London College of Medicine for women. She lectured on health to national health societies and the British County Councils.

To some of my hearers it may seem as if the subject of my paper is rather gruesome, but upon reflection it would appear to be a matter not only of public interest, but of national welfare, that every possible ray of light should be cast

Annesley Kenealy, "The Cholera in Hamburg," in *The Congress of Women: Held in the Women's Building, World's Columbian Exposition, Chicago, U.S.A., 1893.* Chicago: Monarch Book Company, 1894.

on the mysteries and development of that dreaded cholera which worked so much destruction in Hamburg [Germany] during the autumn of 1892, and which appeared to threaten the whole continent of Europe. An account of the rise, the progress and the decline of the epidemic in that city may be instructive and suggestive.

Cholera Streets

Cholera is a disease of which little more is known now than was known when [French novelist] Eugene Sue described it so graphically in the pages of "The Wandering Jew"—description which is thrillingly realistic to anyone who has stood face to face with it. It arises silently and stealthily, doing its dreaded work surely and without pity. Atmosphere and climate conditions affect the development of the germ, for cholera is essentially a germ disease, and impure water and bad sanitation complete the growth. These conditions combined in September, 1892, in Hamburg, and adjoining cities were startled to find the disease so close upon them. As we drove through the streets of the city after a hurried journey from England to the seat of war, if one may so express it, we caught glimpses of the so-called "cholera streets" where the disease arose. The architecture in its antiquity and picturesqueness filled us with admiration; the canals of Stygian blackness, flowing on a level with the lower floors of the houses, reminded us of bits of old Venice, and wanted only the gondoliers to complete the illusion. But while one's artistic senses were satisfied, one's sanitary knowledge rose in revolt against the neglect of all the laws of health as typified in these charming "slums." It would appear that in the towns of Europe it is almost impossible for Art and Hygiene to walk hand in hand. The beautiful "White City" [the name given to the Columbian Exposition] has shown us that they may do so in America. The condemnation of the "cholera streets" is a gain to sanitation, but a terrible sacrifice of art on the altars of the public weal.

The gloomy station at which we alighted was typical of the deserted condition of the city, five Sisters of Mercy and ourselves being the only travelers. To our minds the lapse of duty on the part of the railway employees in forgetting to take our tickets was the strongest possible proof of public demoralization that we saw. That German officialdom could be caught napping was indeed one of the wonders of the cholera epidemic. The city and its streets looked as if under the shadow of a great destiny. Funerals and funeral wreaths, mourners and signs of mourning met us at every corner. The absence of women and children was very conspicuous. It was as if some Pied Piper had passed along and robbed the city of its ornaments. But we learned that forty thousand of the residents had fled on the first mention of cholera, a large proportion of these being women and children.

The Failure of the Authorities to Acknowledge the Presence of the Disease

A picturesque procession, known as the Volunteer Company of Health of Höhenfelde, met us on our route. It consisted of some two dozen men and boys with pails and carboys [containers] of chemicals, whose self-imposed duty it was to go to the places where the disease had been, and thoroughly disinfect and cleanse the rooms and houses. In the early days of the epidemic undoubtedly great confusion reigned; but military discipline soon asserted itself, and out of chaos came order of a most admirable type. I venture to think that few cities of the world would have shown such resource and strength to meet the invasion of so formidable a foe as did Hamburg. The only weak point about the siege was that in the beginning of the epidemic the authorities refused to acknowledge that the enemy was within their gates. Thus the germ was able to take possession of many strongholds which could have been rendered impregnable if proper measures of safety had been adopted sufficiently early. When the fact that cholera had taken possession of the city could no longer be concealed, military cordons were drawn around the infected quarters, ingress and egress being limited to physicians and attendants. But as the proportions of the disease increased, it was found necessary to clear the hospitals of their ordinary patients to make room for the cholera-stricken. In the Eppendorf Hospital, where my sister and I spent some three weeks, there was found accommodation for nearly two thousand patients. This hospital, which is undoubtedly one of the most beautiful in the world, and which closely resembles the Johns Hopkins Hospital of Baltimore, reminded us in its proportions and appearance of a friendly fortress strong to save, and offering a safe refuge to those taking shelter within its walls. The grounds and gardens, full of beautiful flowers and shrubs, the beautiful creepers covering the building, looked, especially at night, when lighted up by electricity, a veritable scene in fairyland. But this likeness was limited to the externals. In the wards there was only the grim realism of suffering and death. In addition to the large wards and partitions, further accommodation was furnished by hospital tents similar to those used in the Franco-Prussian war, which stood picturesquely dotted about in a large waste field adjoining the grounds. These tents grew up almost like the beanstalk of the fairy story—in a single night—and bore testimony to the excellency of the arrangements made by those in authority. Rows of beds stood ready for occupancy, electricity lighted up the interiors as well as the outside, and the tents flying the Red Cross, the emblem of charity and pity, gave one the sense of being in the midst of some military encampment. From a theoretical standpoint, treatment in the open air under canvas would seem a desirable method of treating cholera, and it would appear that thus there would be less danger of the spread of the disease; but, practically, it has been shown that in the cold collapsed condition of the patient, the open air is too depressing. An admirable system of police notification of fresh cases was established, prompt removal being effected by a service of two horsed cabs, which were kept busy night and day. Each vehicle was accompanied by an official, whose duty it was to take the name and address of the stricken patients and furnish this to the hospital, thus affording a ready means of identification in case of death. In the early days of the epidemic, patients were picked up in the streets, unconscious, dying and dead, and were carried to the various hospitals, without any means of tracing their families and friends.

How Cholera Arrived in Hamburg

The disease originated in the shipping quarter, having been brought to Hamburg from the Black Sea by a vessel which successfully concealed the fact that its crew had been stricken by cholera some two months previously. It was natural, therefore, that the sailors and those who go down to the sea in ships should be first attacked. Many foreigners fell victim, whose names never will be known, and whose friends will vainly wait for tidings from and of the lost ones. Curiously enough, my sister was recently asked by a German woman, whom she met in an English country town, whether she could give her any news of a sister who had been lost sight of during the Hamburg epidemic, and who, it was feared, must have shared the common fate. It was by no means unusual for whole families to be taken to the same hospital and distributed in the various wards according to sex and accommodation. Spacious and roomy as these wards were, their capacity was tried to the utmost, the beds, of necessity, being so close that the patients might almost have joined hands round the circumference of the ward. Had not the ventilating and sanitary arrangements been almost perfect, a very serious condition of things would have arisen. The stone floors admirably lent themselves to assidious deluging and mopping with suitable disinfectants. Thus the career of the germ was early cut off.

The appearance of the cholera patient is typical and unlike that of one suffering from any other disease. He is collapsed, with a dusky blackness of skin in many cases, giving the suggestion that his body has been thickly powdered with coal-dust. The normal lines are blackened and deepened, the expression haggard and wan. Listlessness and apathy are expressed in every attitude, and the mental condition, unless the case be complicated with delirium, is distinctly one of lethargy. The rapid emaciation of the body through the draining of the tissue fluids is characteristic only of cholera, and is noticeable in all severe cases. It gives an aged, withered look to the patient, and even the dimpled, rounded limbs of the young child will lose contour, and become wrinkled and shrunk in the space of a few hours. A consuming thirst is so great as to almost absorb all other sensations, and results in the enormous consumption of liquids and in part restores the loss of the fluid components of the body through the disease. This thirst is constant and unrelievable, and was one of the difficulties of the situation. Hard pressed as we were to supply the bare needs of our patients, it was most pathetic to be frequently obliged to ignore for a space their entreaties for drink of any and every kind, and to note the wistful, thirsty eyes of the occupants as we passed their beds to supply some one whose needs were greater. The tight clutch of baby hands on mugs and glasses told us how real was the desire for liquid. Often in the midst of our duties we would hear a small thud on the ground, followed by patter of little feet that scarcely knew how to walk, setting out on a small voyage of discovery and investigation into the contents of bottles and jugs that stood in the wards. It has been said that a large proportion of cholera patients die of fear, but I believe this conclusion to have been reached from observations made in India. Doubtless the nervous, highly-strung Hindoo [sic] would see in the invasion of cholera the finger of fate, against which he would believe medical skill to be quite powerless. . . . It frequently occurred to us that the choleraic condition killed all natural emotion. Little sisters side by side in bed, one would die, and the other would take no notice and feel no fear. Older children would see their mothers carried dead from the wards, and would watch the procession as of something afar off that had no relation to them. The rapid succession of patients was most bewildering—not, unfortunately, because of recovery, but because of deaths. Almost before we had time to know the faces of our patients they were removed to the mortuary, and others were ready to take the vacant beds. Cholera spares neither sex nor age. Our patients ranged from the baby at the breast to those who had fulfilled their three-score years and ten [the span of life, or seventy years]. The fight was by no means always to the strong, and victory not at all necessarily to those of robust nature. Treatment consisted chiefly of venous injections of warm salt and water, combined with hot, stimulating baths and packs, but the general consensus of medical opinion at Hamburg was that no remedy could in any sense be relied on. Our own experience bears out that which has been aptly said regarding the disease, that "if the patient be strong enough, or can in any way be assisted to survive the attack, it might be said he was cured of cholera, but it was the man who lived, and not that the cholera was killed." Prevention is the only cure. Epidemics are nature's health officers, and they do their work efficiently if they are sufficiently serious to impress themselves upon the public mind. Slowly and by degrees, as malarial and deadly spots in India are drained and sanitated, the outbreaks of cholera are fewer and less serious. Disease is a foe that recedes as the missionaries of health advance. Gradually, as more light is thrown on the science of hygiene, the legions of microbes ever lurking in darkness and dirt are stifled in their growth and become weaker and weaker. The insanitation of India, the starvation and misery of Russia, are a standing menace to the peoples of Europe, and so long as these exist, each year we will have to gird up our strength to meet the foe, and shall have to grapple hard to keep him to his own quarters—the quarters of dirt and uncivilization.

In these days of express speed we have many advantages. The railroad and steamboat bring us into relation with the uttermost ends of the earth and the peoples thereof, but we must not lose sight of the fact that at the same time we are brought into contact with the moral and physical diseases of all these different peoples.

What Hamburg Could Have Done to Prevent Cholera

The "sins of Hamburg" were great, and eventually found her out. Nature had dealt very gently with her breaches of the eternal laws of health. Thirteen comparatively mild epidemics had failed to suggest to the city authorities the necessity of putting their house in order. The Elbe water was still supplied in all its native and imported impurity, and then came the fourteenth warning, sadder, sharper and effectual, and Hamburg has risen to the occasion. From her commercial position and harbor accommodations Hamburg is peculiarly open to the importation of foreign diseases, and it is only by keeping her hearths well garnished and the city household in health that she can afford to admit suspicious visitors. It is a matter of menace and regret that she did not enforce compulsory cremation during the cholera epidemic. A beautiful crematorium, hitherto practically unused, stood all through the epidemic as a silent but eloquent monument to the prejudices of the people. In certain conditions of the soil a cholera body is more dangerous to the community when below than when above the ground, and it is much to be feared that a heavy day of reckoning must come when it is remembered that countless thousands of cholera corpses are giving their noxious emanations to the atmosphere of Hamburg.

A physician, recently writing in a professional paper, makes use of the following astonishing statement that cholera gives a new lease of life to the sufferer. This may be so if he means us to understand some transcendental lease in another sphere, but if he alludes to a lease here below, I cannot but think that the most of us should object to the terms of the agreement. There is no question but that, in the marvelous cleaning up of Europe that has followed the cholera scare, there will be found new leases of life to whole nations consequent to improved health conditions. Let me commend the system to Chicago. In my stay here during the World's Fair I have noted whole rows of "cholera streets," which have not even the excuse of being artistic.

Tracts were distributed broadcast among the patients in the German hospitals persuading them in solemn language that the cholera epidemic was a merciful dispensation on the part of a wise Providence, and that the gentle chastisement had been sent as a reminder that their ways of life were evil. But not a word was said of the evil ways of the authorities of the city, who allowed the water supply to become so polluted that "death in the cup" might be taken more as a statement of fact than as a poetical exaggeration.

In conclusion let me offer a deserved tribute to the energy, the self-denial and devotion of Hamburg and her sons and daughters during the period of suffering. Nurses, physicians and attendants worked with a singleness of purpose and for-getfulness of self. Much illness arose and many deaths oc-curred in the ranks, but all stood by their guns with a courage that was one of the most hopeful beacons at a time when en-couraging signals were much needed.

Truly "unhappy Hamburg" has been the scapegoat for sanitary sins. She was far in advance of most continental cities in sanitation, notwithstanding she was singled out and other much worse offenders were passed by unharmed. But the warning has been to all to gird up their loins and prepare their strongholds to meet attacks from an enemy so mighty and subtle and mysterious that his coming is always stealthy, and, as it were, in the dead of night.

The American Colonies Deal with Public Health Concerns

Elizabeth C. Tandy

The first settlers arrived in the New World often malnourished and in a weakened state according to Elizabeth C. Tandy, the author of the selection included here. Once in their new environment they spread disease and also fell victim to the diseases of the Native Americans with whom they came in contact. Tandy's article focuses on a time span of 155 years during which the individual colonies took measures to stem the spread of disease. These measures were among the nation's earliest attempts at public health.

One of the classic measures of combating contagious disease was quarantine, or isolation of the ill. Colonial rules governing quarantine were loose at first but took on greater stringency as the colonies grew. As Tandy points out, the early quarantines were extended to land as well as to ships at port and included not only the ill but also those who came into contact with the sick. Inoculation was another method used by the colonists to stem the spread of diseases, especially smallpox. Initially, inoculation was controversial, with some colonists favoring it and others vehemently opposed. By 1777, however, inoculation was viewed as a necessary preventive measure with none other than George Washington ordering the inoculation of his army at Valley Forge.

Elizabeth Tandy wrote her article on the history of quarantine and inoculation for the committee on dispensary development for the United Hospital Fund, New York City.

Elizabeth C. Tandy, "Local Quarantine and Inoculation for Smallpox in the American Colonies (1620–1775)," *American Journal of Public Health*, March 13, 1923, pp. 203–207. Reproduced by permission of American Public Health Association.

The colonization of America was a bitter fight with disease and death from the very moment the resolute emigrants set foot on the little vessels which were to carry them on their long voyage. In crowded, insanitary quarters, poorly supplied with food and medicine, the prospective colonists spent dreary and seasick months on shipboard. Some contagious or infectious disease usually appeared. Francis Blackwell, a leading Puritan of Amsterdam, lost two-thirds of the one hundred and eighty fellow emigrants who were herded in his small vessel bound for Virginia (1618). At a later date, William Penn (1682) lost thirty of his company by smallpox. John Winthrop wrote to his wife, November 29, 1630, of the many deaths which occurred during that first terrible winter in the Plymouth settlement. "We conceive that this disease grew out of ill diet at sea and proved infectious." Bad food, exposure and disease brought an enfeebled group of settlers to the New World.

The early settlers discounted their weakened condition. They recognized the necessity of cooperation in time of sickness as well as in time of health. There is no record to show that one of them failed to help a brother in time of distress. In the New England colonies the newcomers extended this conception of brotherhood to include the natives. Of the year 1634 [William] Bradford [governor of Plymouth colony] writes:

"This spring also, those Indians about their trading house there fell sick of the small poxe and died most miserably; ... The condition of the people was so lamentable and they fell down so generally of this disease as they were in the end not able to help one another ... those of the English house (though at first they were afraid of the infection) yet seeing this woefull and sadd condition; and hearing their pitifull cries and lamentations, they had compasion on them and daily fetched them wood and water, and made them fires, got them victuals whilst they lived, and buried them when they died. For very few of them escaped, notwithstanding what they did for them to the hazard of themselves. . . . But by the marvelous providence of God not one of the English was so much as sicke, or in the least measure tainted with the disease, though they daily did them offices for many weeks together."

John Winthrop [governor of Massachusetts colony] writes of the same epidemic in his Journal, February 1st, (1634).

"Such of the Indians' children as were left were taken by the English. Most whereof did die of the pox soon after."

The cooperation of these people in a crisis is perhaps characteristic of a pioneer society. The fear of contagion was great. Deliverance was considered as due to "God's Wonderworking Providence." Early epidemics were met by the setting aside of days for humiliation and prayer. Governments and individuals made covenants with the Lord. These seem to have been entered into about the time the pestilence had run its course, at any rate immediately thereafter "the airs" were wont "to lighten and the sick to improve."

Quarantine

The idea of quarantine was at first directed toward disease which entered by sea. The earliest instance is probably that of the quarantine against ships from Barbadoes in 1647. Colonial records show constant effort to minimize the amount of disease entering from foreign sources. Statutes directed toward this type of protection were passed by the General Assemblies and received the sanction of the crown at an early date in almost every colony.

The concept of local quarantine and isolation was evidently a later development than the idea of foreign exclusion. Evidence of local attempt is not recorded prior to the sixties. The first group action for the exclusion of contagious disease by land quarantine is found in the Town Records of East Hampton, L. I., under the date March 2, 1662. It reads as follows:

"It is ordered that no Indian shall come to towne into the street after sufficient notice upon penalty of 5 s. [shillings] or be whipped until they be free from small poxe; but that they may come where they have corne on the back side and call; and if any English or Indian servant shall go to their wigwams they shall suffer the same punishment."

Acting under the very general authority given by the Governor and the Company of Massachusetts Bay, the Salem selectmen passed their first ordinance in 1678:

"It is ordered that William Stacy who is sick of the small pox doeth not presume to Come abroad till three weeks after this date be expired and that he be very careful yt when yt time be expired he shift his Clothes ans doe not frequent any Company till he be wholly cure of that infection."

Colonial local quarantines were for many years founded upon vague authority. The selectmen of Massachusetts had the most definite grant of power. They based their early regulations upon the edict of the Governor and the Company of Massachusetts Bay, dated March 12, 1635.

"Whereas particular townes have many things which concerne only themselves, and the ordering of their own affairs . . . it is therefore ordered that the freemen of every towne, or the major part of them, shall have power to . . . make such orders as may concerne the well ordering of their owne townes, not repugnant to the laws and orders here established by the General Court."

Further authority was not secured in this colony until the passage of the act of 1701–1702 which related to land and maritime quarantine. Under the first part of this law the selectmen of the towns were, "empowered to take care and make effectual provision in the best manner" they could for the preservation of the inhabitants "by removing and placing such sick or infected persons to and in separate houses, and by providing nurses, tendance and other assistance and necessaries for them at the expense of the parties themselves, their parents or masters (if able) or otherwise at the charge of the town or place whereto they belonged." In case it happened persons were "visited with sickness in any other town or place than that" whereto they belonged and occasioned charge to such town, the selectmen were to lay the charge before the justices of the peace of the town of which they were inhabitants and the justices were empowered to adjust and pay the accounts. Charge for care during sickness of indigent persons who had no settlement in the province was to be paid out of the colonial treasury. Power was given to the justices of the peace to impress "convenient housing, lodging, nursing, tendance, and other necessaries" for the relief of the sick.

Alerting the Community

This act of 1701–1702 was followed by "An Act to Prevent Persons from Concealing the Small Pox" passed in 1731. It required that when any person visited with the smallpox in any town should become aware of the infection the head of the house should acquaint the selectmen of the fact and also hang out a pole bearing a red flag of prescribed dimensions. The flag was to continue until in the judgment of the selectmen the house was thoroughly aired and cleansed. The penalty for breaking quarantine was a fine of 50 pounds. With this legislation as authority, the selectmen of the towns of Massachusetts drew a prodigious number of quarantine warrants, impressed houses and nurses for infected individuals, and provided medical care. In 1764–1765 the assembly authorized the selectmen to appoint or impress guards for any house wherein any person might be visited with the smallpox, and directed that guards so appointed should prevent all persons from going in or coming out of infected houses without a license from the selectmen.

The next colony to secure legislative authority for local quarantine was South Carolina. Under a law entitled "An Act for the Better Preventing of the Spreading of the Small Pox in Charleston," dated 1738, it was enacted that when any person in any house or plantation discovered himself to be infected with the smallpox the master of the house should immediately affix an advertisement of the fact to the post on the nearest public road and a similar advertisement in the nearest parish house or church. Failure to perform this duty was punished by a fine of 50 pounds. Justices were empowered to impress guards and directed to place them on all houses where anyone was sick with the smallpox.

The colony of New York protected itself in time of epidemic without legislative authority up to the year 1755. The method of protection initiated in East Hampton was frequently invoked. An instance of the grant of power to the selectmen by the citizens occurs in the Huntington Town Records for the year 1771:

> "It was voted that the Trustees should have full Power to make any Prudential rules and orders in the Town Concerning the small pox and any other thing that shall seem to be needful."

Legislative authority for local quarantine was secured by an act supplementary to the maritime quarantine law of 1755.

Pennsylvania was without authority for local quarantine until well after the War for Independence. Indeed, in the colonial statutes of Pennsylvania smallpox was not a disease for which even seaboard quarantine might be established.

The principles of local quarantine were fairly well established early in the colonial period. The first regulations were passed by the citizens in town meeting. These were based upon indefinite grants of power. Statutory authority was secured somewhat later.

Quarantines were adopted whenever any plainly contagious malady became prevalent. Most of the colonial quarantines were directed toward the control of smallpox. Methods of segregation were seldom, if ever, successful in arresting the progress of the epidemic disease.

Inoculation

The next important development was that of inoculation against smallpox. This form of preventive medicine was introduced into colonial society about 1721. It resulted in much excitement and opposition. Although inoculation was a success from the first, those voluntarily contracting the disease were considered a menace. In 1722 the Reverend [Lee] Massey took as his text, "So went Satan forth from the presence of the Lord, and smote Job with sore boils from the sole of his foot unto his crown," and asserted that the Devil was the first inoculator and poor Job was his first patient. With the change in attitude the sermon gave rise to a verse which appeared in the *Monthly Miscellany* for March, 1774:

"We are told by one of the black robe The Devil inoculated Job. Suppose 'tis true, what he does tell, Pray, Neighbors, did not Job do well?"

Cotton Mather [the Puritan minister], an ardent advocate of the protective method, permitted individuals to undergo inoculation in his house. While he was harboring such a person an indignant citizen threw a grenade through the window. As late as 1774, a hospital in Salem was burned for fear that it would be turned into an inoculation hospital. Progressive individuals, however, in spite of popular disapproval, were anxious to avoid the full virulence of the disease. They arranged for the inoculation of themselves and their entire families. Inoculating hospitals sprang up to serve them in many localities, and at length the first general hospital known to have existed for this purpose in New England was opened on Cat Island, near Salem, in the year 1773.

Orders restricting inoculation were first of a local character. For the most part they recognized the right of individuals to decide for themselves whether they should undergo inoculation, and charged them that they "should not come or walk abroad in the streets, lanes or alleys within the towns until their incisions" were "well Cleansed and Healed." Other orders defined the limits within which inoculating hospitals would not be permitted. It was customary to locate them in unfrequented neighborhoods or on islands.

Colonial legislation in regard to inoculation first appeared in the colony of South Carolina. In the year 1738 the assembly enacted that nobody in Charleston or within two miles of the city limits should inoculate any person or permit himself to be inoculated under penalty of a fine of 500 pounds.

Massachusetts legislation was at first likewise directed toward the protection of the citizens of its principal city. An act of 1763–1764 prohibited any person from inoculating or being inoculated in the city of Boston. Penalty for violation was 50 pounds. After thirty families were known to be visited with the distemper at one time, and the selectmen gave public notice that they had no hope of stopping progress of the epidemic, inoculation was formally permitted.

Early New York legislation in certain districts restricted inoculation. The first law, passed in 1772, prohibited the practice within the distance of a quarter of a mile of a dwelling house, public road or landing place within Westchester, Dutchess and Orange counties. Every offense was to be penalized by a fine of five pounds and costs. Nothing in the law was to be construed to prevent any family from being inoculated within their own dwellings. The next year an act was passed to repeal this law in so far as it applied to the borough and town of Westchester. The inhabitants of the district judged that the law "had a bad tendency." The same year a law was passed to regulate the practice in the city of Albany. License was required of persons intending to use any house or building within the city as an inoculating hospital. Nothing in the act was to deprive or prevent any person from inoculating individuals or his own family within his own private dwelling.

Pennsylvania, with characteristic disregard of the contagious nature of smallpox, passed no colonial laws in regard to inoculation.

By the end of the colonial period the practice of inoculation had passed through the period of fiery opposition and been accepted as a comparatively effective method of avoiding the dire results of the actual disease. While few statutes deprived individuals of the right to be inoculated within their own dwellings, the long period of isolation and the better facilities for medical care served to make inoculation more popular in the hospitals than at home. Whole families, joined by numbers of friends, frequently repaired to the inoculating house and enjoyed one another's society during the long period of seclusion. Many of the romances of the later colonial days were initiated in the propinquity these hospitals afforded.

Very early in the War for Independence smallpox became epidemic in the colonial army. Dr. [Benjamin] Church, surgeon general, soon issued orders for the inoculation of the army in Massachusetts. In February, 1777, General [George] Washington wrote to Congress that it was impossible to keep the smallpox from spreading through the whole army, and that he was determined not only to inoculate the troops but to order that the recruits be inoculated at the time of enlistment. The autumn of 1777 saw the general inoculation of the colonial army at Valley Forge.

Organizing for Protection

In the period that intervened between the landing of the Pilgrims and the drafting of the Constitution for the United States Government there was considerable change in ideas regarding the protection of public health from communicable disease. Colonies which started with prayers to the Lord for deliverance and the promiscuous spreading of infection came to recognize the highly contagious and infectious nature of a few diseases. Restrictive quarantine laws imposing heavy fines were enacted in most of the provinces. Administrative machinery of a simple sort was developed. Public health protection through compulsory inoculation for smallpox was established to apply to army recruits. The period shows a great advance in community organization for self-protection.

It is notable that advance in health protection was not by sweeping intercolonial legislation. Every step was undertaken in the face of strong opposition. Every new development had to be put through by each individual community as the result of fight against deep-rooted prejudice. Habits of individual indifference and reliance upon divine intervention rather than scientific precaution were slow in dying. The advanced stage of health protection which the colonies had reached by the time of the War for Independence testifies to the courage, tenacity and clear insightedness of a few leaders, conspicuously Mather and [Benjamin] Franklin, but also intelligent physicians and hardheaded country squires, far more than such progress indicates the open-mindedness of the entire group of colonial inhabitants.

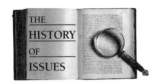

CHAPTER 2

Public Health in the United States Through the Mid-Twentieth Century

Chapter Preface

Although the first attempt by the federal government to control public health began with the establishment of the Marine Hospital Service in 1798 it was the individual states and cities that continued to bear the responsibility for the health and well-being of the citizenry well into the 1800s. In the mid-1800s, for example, the Massachusetts Sanitary Commission launched a survey of the state to ascertain its health problems and make recommendations for a public health code. The findings of the commission were compiled by Lemuel Shattuck and called for the formation of boards of health at the local and state levels. Although the recommendations of the commission never became law they did establish the foundation for a public health code. The public health code as envisioned by Shattuck was wide-ranging: It called for compiling statistics on specific diseases such as cholera and pneumonia to dictating the location and care of burial grounds.

The protection of the health and welfare of the population was of greatest concern in the nation's ports and leading economic centers. The reasons were obvious. Wealth in nineteenth-century America was being generated in urban centers such as New York, Boston, Chicago, and San Francisco. These cities, located as they are at major transit hubs, were often afflicted with outbreaks of contagious diseases. It became imperative therefore to find ways to combat disease over the long term and not merely respond to a crisis. This imperative gave rise to the sanitarian movement. One aspect of the movement was the improvement of the environment. In New York City, the nation's most important port and financial center, engineers constructed public works such as sewer and water supply systems and city officials secured control over the water that flowed into the metropolis. The nation's first totally independent public health department came into being in

New York in 1866. In a short period of time medical professionals and reformers working within urban health departments were responding to a new public health need: the care and education of immigrants. Public health nurses fanned out into immigrant neighborhoods to teach newcomers the importance of good hygiene. Boards of health took a special interest in the welfare and health of young children.

Outbreaks of disease continued to challenge the public health system well into the twentieth century, however. The 1918–19 Spanish influenza pandemic is a case in point. As the flu skipped and hopped across the United States, afflicting terrible losses on some cities and towns while leaving some untouched, it became apparent that the nation lacked a coherent way of dealing with epidemics. The following chapter discusses this subject and the rise of boards of health, the emergence of government agencies (such as the Food and Drug Administration (FDA)) to oversee the public health, and the extent to which a board of health is empowered to protect the public.

The Marine Hospital Service Is a Federal Effort in Public Health

U.S. National Library of Medicine

The treatment of diseases in colonial America was limited and ideas about how communities should respond to the threat of diseases were elementary. Doctors and governmental leaders of the 1700s concentrated their efforts on protecting the population through quarantine and inoculation. All efforts were at the local level.

The nation's earliest federally organized public health system began in 1798 with the passage of the Act for the Relief of Sick and Disabled Seamen. The act, signed into law by President John Adams, aimed to protect and care for merchant seamen who often arrived in the nation's ports ill and without family members to care for them. Since public hospitals were limited in the number of patients they could admit and townspeople reluctant to take in sick naval personnel out of fear of contagion, a special fund was established to build marine hospitals especially for the sailors. This event marked the beginning of the U.S. Public Health Service (PHS). The following selection, written to mark the one hundredth anniversary of the PHS, describes the evolution of the Marine Hospital Service and its work from its beginnings in the late 1700s to the present day.

Early History

The PHS [Public Health Service] grew out of a need for healthy seamen in our infant republic, which relied so much on the sea for trade and security. These seamen traveled widely, often became sick at sea, and then, away from their

U.S. National Library of Medicine, "Introduction: Two Centuries of Health Promotion," January 2005.

homes and families, could not find adequate health care in the port cities they visited or would overburden the meager public hospitals then in existence. Since they came from all the new states and former colonies, and could get sick anywhere, their health care became a national or Federal problem. A loose network of marine hospitals, mainly in port cities, was established by Congress in 1798 to care for these sick and disabled seamen, and was called the Marine Hospital Service (MHS).

The Federal Government had only three executive departments then to administer all Federal programs—State, Treasury, and War. The MHS was placed under the Revenue Marine Division of the Treasury Department. Funds to pay physicians and build marine hospitals were appropriated by taxing American seamen 20 cents a month. This was one of the first direct taxes enacted by the new republic and the first medical insurance program in the United States. The monies were collected from ship masters by the customs collectors in different U.S. ports.

The President was granted the authority to appoint the directors of these hospitals, but later allowed the customs collectors to do it. The appointments thus became influenced by local politics and practices. Often times hospitals were built to meet political rather than medical needs. Each hospital was managed independently and the Treasury Department had no supervisory mechanism to centralize or coordinate their activity. For example, the report of a Congressional commission formed to investigate the MHS stated in 1851 that the "hospital at Mobile [Alabama] is as distinct and different from that at Norfolk [Virginia] or New Orleans as if it were a hotel and the other a hospital. . . ."

Lack of money, in addition to the lack of any supervisory authority, was another major problem for the MHS. The demand for medical services far exceeded the funds available. For that reason sailors with chronic or incurable conditions were excluded from the hospitals and a four-month limit was placed on hospital care for the rest. Additional funds had to be appropriated constantly from Congress in order to maintain the Service and to build the hospitals. Because of these problems Congress was forced to act and in 1870 reorganized the MHS from a loose network of locally-controlled hospitals to a centrally-controlled national agency with its own administrative staff, administration and headquarters in Washington, D.C.

MHS Becomes a Bureau of the Treasury Department and Broadens Its Scope

Through this reorganization, the MHS became a separate bureau of the Treasury Department under the supervision of the Supervising Surgeon, who was appointed by the Secretary of the Treasury. The title of the central administrator was changed to Supervising Surgeon General in 1875 and to Surgeon General in 1902. Additional money to fund the reorganized Service was appropriated by raising the hospital tax on seamen from twenty to forty cents per month. The money collected was deposited in a separate MHS fund.

Taxing seamen to fund the MHS was abolished in 1884. From 1884 to 1906 the cost of maintaining the marine hospitals was paid from the proceeds of a tonnage tax on vessels entering the United States, and from 1906 to 1981, when the Public Health Service hospitals were closed, by direct appropriations from Congress.

The 1870 reorganization also changed the general character of the Service. It became national in scope and military in outlook and organization. Medical officers, called surgeons, were required to pass entrance examinations and wear uniforms. In 1889, when the Commissioned Corps was formally recognized by legislative action, the medical officers were given title and pay corresponding to Army and Navy grades. Physicians who passed the examinations were appointed to the general service, rather than to a particular hospital, and were assigned wherever needed. The goal was to create a professional, mobile, health corps, free as possible from political favoritism and patronage, and able to deal with the new health needs of a rapidly growing and industrializing nation.

Epidemics of contagious diseases, such as small pox, yellow fever, and cholera, had devastating effects throughout the 19th century. They killed many people, spread panic and fear, disrupted government, and caused Congress to enact laws to stop their importation and spread. As a result of these new laws, the functions of the MHS were expanded greatly beyond the medical relief of the sick seamen to include the supervision of national quarantine (ship inspection and disinfection), the medical inspection of immigrants, the prevention of interstate spread of disease, and general investigations in the field of public health, such as that of yellow fever epidemics.

To help diagnose infectious diseases among passengers of incoming ships, the MHS established in 1887 a small bacteriology laboratory, called the Hygienic Laboratory, at the marine hospital on Staten Island, New York. That laboratory later moved to Washington, D.C., and became the National Institutes of Health, the largest biomedical research organization in the world.

To better consolidate these increased functions of the MHS, including medical research, and give them legal powers, Congress passed an act in 1902 which expanded the scientific research work at the Hygienic Laboratory and gave it a definite budget. The bill also required the Surgeon General to organize annual conferences of local and national health officials in order to coordinate better state and national public health activities, and changed the name of the MHS to the Public Health and Marine Hospital Services (PHMHS) to reflect its broader scope.

The PHMHS was not the only government agency engaged in health-related work. The enforcement of the pure food and drugs law, passed in 1906, was placed in the hands of the Bureau of Chemistry of the Department of Agriculture. The Federal inspection of meats entering interstate commerce, also mandated by law in 1906, was done by the Bureau of Animal Industry of the Department of Agriculture. The Bureau of the Census was authorized in 1902 to collect vital statistics—data relating to health and disease from around the country.

Efforts to Consolidate Public Health Services

Efforts were made during the early decades of the 20th century by both political parties and by people inside and outside of government concerned with the nation's health to combine public health-related work being done by various Federal agencies, but they were unsuccessful in Congress. The act of August 14, 1912, changed the name of the PHMHS to the Public Health Service [PHS] and further broadened its powers by authorizing investigations into human diseases (such as, tuberculosis, hookworm, malaria, and leprosy), sanitation, water supplies and sewage disposal, but went no further.

Real consolidation began in June 1939, when the PHS was transferred by President Franklin D. Roosevelt to the newly created Federal Security Agency (FSA), which combined a number of New Deal government agencies and services related to health, education, and welfare. Over 140 years of association between the PHS and the Treasury Department came to an end. All of the laws affecting the functions of the services were also consolidated for the first time in the Public Health Services Act of 1944.

The FSA was a noncabinet-level agency whose programs grew to such size and scope that, in 1953, President [Dwight D.] Eisenhower submitted a reorganization plan to Congress which called for the dissolution of the FSA and the transfer of all its responsibilities to a newly created Department of Health,

Education, and Welfare (HEW). A major objective of this reorganization was to ensure that the important areas of health, education, and social security be represented in the President's cabinet. In 1979, HEW's educational tasks were transferred to the new Department of Education and the remaining divisions of HEW were reorganized as the Department of Health and Human Services (HHS).

Throughout all of these reorganizations which have shaped, defined, and established the PHS in its present place in the Federal Government, and which have spanned nearly two centuries, the PHS has never lost sight of its primary goal—providing health care for those with special needs. From the care of sick and disabled sailors the PHS has extended its activities to other groups with special needs (such as, the American Indians, the Alaska Natives, migrant workers, Federal prisoners, and refugees), and to the nation as a whole.

The duties and functions of the PHS have expanded to include disease control and prevention, biomedical research, regulation of food and drugs, mental health and drug abuse, health care delivery, and international health.

The Shattuck Report Calls for Improving the Health of Bostonians, 1850

Lemuel Shattuck

In 1850, the legislature of Massachusetts surveyed the sanitary conditions of the state's towns and cities and issued a report on the findings. The statistical survey was carried out by Lemuel Shattuck, who gave his name to the report and recommended the formation of boards of health at the state and local levels. The legislature did not adopt Shattuck's broad-ranging proposal, however. It was not until the twentieth century that Lemuel Shattuck's concepts of public health were put into practice. Nevertheless, his recommendations became the foundation of the sanitation movement in the United States and his proposed laws were the first attempt to write a comprehensive public health code.

The following selection contains excerpts from Shattuck's 1850 report. The recommendations call for compiling information on diseases, the treatment of the insane, the management of burial sites, the health and welfare of seamen, the treatment of the health and hygiene of immigrants, and more.

XXIII. We recommend *that local Boards of Health, and other persons interested, endeavor to ascertain, by exact observation, the effect of mill-ponds, and other collections or streams of water, and of their rise and fall, upon the health of the neighboring inhabitants.*

We have seen that the question involved in this recommendation has had an historical interest; though it seems of

Lemuel Shattuck, "Report of a General Plan for the Promotion of General and Public Health Devised, Prepared and Recommended by the Commissioners Appointed under a Resolution of the Legislature of Massachusetts Relating to the Sanitary Survey of the State," April 26, 1850. http://biotech.law.lsu.edu/cphl.

late to be almost entirely forgotten. The streams at the water-falls, in all parts of the Commonwealth, are obstructed in their courses for manufacturing purposes; and if cases of fever or other disease occur in the neighborhood, the people have generally attributed them to some uncontrollable agency; while possibly, perhaps, they may arise from causes which their own hands have created, and which are capable of removal. It is then a question of permanent interest and importance. If mill-ponds, or stagnant waters of any kind, or places where they have existed, produce disease under certain conditions, it should be known, and certain other conditions should be provided, under which they may be permitted without injury, and without which they should not be permitted at all. . . .

XXIV. We recommend *that the local Boards of Health provide for periodical house-to-house visitation, for the prevention of epidemic diseases, and for other sanitary purposes.*

The approach of many epidemic diseases is often fore-shadowed by some derangement in the general health; and, if properly attended to at that time, the fatal effects may be prevented. This is especially proper in regard to cholera and dysentery. The premonitory symptoms of cholera are seldom absent; and if these are seasonably observed and properly treated, the disease is controllable. There are few diseases over which curative measures have less, and few over which preventive measures have greater power. This well-known characteristic of the disease led persons in many places in England, during last year, to organize a system of house-to-house visitation, by which every family, sick or well, in a given district, was visited daily by some authorized person, whether invited or not; and every inmate who had the least symptom of the disease received advice and treatment. . . .

XXV. We recommend *that measures be taken to ascertain the amount of sickness suffered in different localities; and among persons of different classes, professions, and occupations.*

Every person is liable to sickness. The extent of that liability, however, varies in different places and circumstances, and in the same place and circumstances in different ages and seasons. It has some, though not an exact, relation to mortality. . . .

There are several reasons why this subject should be fully and carefully investigated, and that exact facts in relation to different populations, existing under different circumstances, should be known. We shall allude to two principal ones only:

1. *It would subserve a pecuniary purpose.* The wealth of a country consists in its capacity for labor. That people who enjoy the greatest vital force,—the highest degree of health,—and apply it most skilfully to the production of wealth, are the most wealthy. It is their capital, their means of subsistence. Persons who sustain a low vitality only, generally have little skill to apply what they possess, contribute little or nothing to the general welfare, and may, and often actually do, become a public burden. This is one view. . . .

2. *It would subserve a sanitary purpose,* and show the exact condition of the people. Some interesting facts on this subject are already known. The Manchester [England] Statistical Society have given the average number of days of sickness annually suffered by each of the operatives engaged in various branches of industry, from which it appears that, in the Staffordshire potteries, under the age of 60, it is 9.03 days; in the silk mills, 7.08 days; in the woolen mills, 7.08 days; in the flax mills, 5.09 days; in the cotton mills at Glasgow [Scotland], 5.06 days; among the East India Company [British overseas trading company] servants, 5.04 days; among laborers in the dock-yards, 5.38 days; in the Lancashire [England] cotton mills, 5.35 days; and for those under 16, 3.14 days. . . .

These are some of the interesting results of the investigations made in England and Scotland, relating to sickness. How far they are applicable to this country we have not the means of knowing accurately. Some have supposed that the proportion of sickness to health is greater in Massachusetts than in England, but others are of a different opinion. The observations already made are too limited and imperfect to found thereon any correct opinion. If the rule of doubling the annual mortality per cent. be applied to obtain the rate of sickness, it will appear that 5.06 per cent. of the population, or 5,787 persons of both sexes, have on the average been constantly sick, in Boston, for the last nine years. By the same rule, in a country town of an average healthy standard, containing 2,000 inhabitants, 60 will constantly be sick. This seems a large proportion or amount of sickness, but it may nevertheless be true, where those in infancy and old age are included.

This subject is of vast consequence. It would be extremely interesting and useful to know the amount of sickness in the families, and among persons of the various professions and occupations,—the farmers, the mechanics, the manufacturers, and others,—and how far it differs in different places and under different circumstances. . . .

XXVI. We recommend *that measures be taken to ascertain the amount of sickness suffered, among the scholars who attend the public schools and other seminaries of learning in the Commonwealth.*

It has recently been recommended that the science of physiology be taught in the public schools; and the recommendation should be universally approved and carried into effect as soon as persons can be found capable of teaching it. Sanitary science is intimately connected with physiology, and deserves equal and even greater commendation as a branch of education. Every child should be taught, early in life, that, to preserve his own life and his own health and the lives and health of others, is one of his most important and constantly abiding *duties*. By obeying certain laws, or performing certain acts, his life and health may be preserved; by disobedience, or performing certain other acts, they will both be destroyed. By knowing and avoiding the causes of disease, disease itself will be avoided, and he may enjoy health and live; by ignorance of these causes and exposure to them, he may contract disease, ruin his health, and die. Every thing connected with wealth, happiness and long life depend upon *health*; and even the great duties of morals and religion are performed more acceptably in a healthy than in a sickly condition. . . .

XXVII. We recommend *that every city and town in the State be* required *to provide means for the periodical vaccination of the inhabitants.*

The small-pox is a terrific disease; but it is almost entirely shorn of its terrors by the preventive remedy of vaccination. If a person is not vaccinated, there is more than two chances to one, that, if exposed, he will take the disease; but, if properly vaccinated, there is scarcely one chance in five hundred. Hence the importance of this preventive measure, and the guilt of neglecting it. . . .

Under existing circumstances, it becomes the special duty of every person to protect himself against this disease. Any one who permits himself to be sick with it, is as justly chargeable with ignorance, negligence or guilt, as he who leaves his house open to be entered and pillaged by robbers, known to be in the neighborhood. And upon that state, city, or town, which does not interpose its legal authority to exterminate the disease, should rest the responsibility, as must rest the consequences, of permitting the destruction of the lives and the health of its citizens. . . .

XXIX. We recommend *that nuisances endangering human life or health, prevented, destroyed, or mitigated.*

Nuisances are divided, in law, into two principal classes:

1. Those which affect the community, or the public, denominated *public nuisances*; and 2. Those which affect the rights or injure the property of individuals, denominated *private nuisances*. Some nuisances have a disagreeable and some a pecuniary character only. Others, a vital or sanitary character. The last class, only, immediately concerns this recommendation.

A street, highway, or bridge, is common property, and any obstruction, pit-hole, or defect, which endangers the lives of travellers, is a nuisance. Horses, cattle, swine, or other animals, going at large in such street or highway, may also be a nuisance. Locomotive steam carriages, steamboats, or other vehicles, or stationary steam engines, may become so by the manner in which they are managed. The manufacture, storage; and use of gunpowder and fireworks may be a nuisance, if within the neighborhood of living beings, since they endanger life. Gas, camphine, and other burning fluids, are often destructive of life. These and all other nuisances of a sanitary character, which often occasion direct accidental injury or death, should be so regulated as not to become dangerous to health and life. . . .

XXXII. We recommend *that the authority now vested in justices of the peace, relating to insane and idiotic persons, not arrested or indicted for crime, be transferred to the local Boards of Health.*

By the present laws of the State, no insane or idiotic person, other than paupers, can be committed to any hospital or place of confinement, except on complaint, in writing, before two justices of the peace, or some police court. Paupers may be committed by the overseers of the poor. By these proceedings, this unfortunate class of persons appear on the records as criminals, while they are guilty of no crime, unless the possession of an unsound mind be considered one. A sanitary question, merely, is often the only one presented in such cases, and it has occurred to us that the local Boards of Health would be the proper tribunals before whom they should be brought, and by whom they should be disposed of. It may be supposed that such Boards will be better acquainted, generally, with the medical jurisprudence of insanity, than justices of the peace; and their decisions will be, more than those of criminal courts, in accordance with the spirit of humanity which has been extended to that class of persons.

XXXIII. We recommend *that the general management of cemeteries and other places of burial, and of the interment of the dead, be regulated by the local Boards of Health.*

The Revised Statutes provide that towns may grant money for burial-grounds, and that Boards of Health "shall make all regulations which they may judge necessary for the interment of the dead, and respecting burying-grounds in their towns." This is all the legal authority that is necessary for the purposes of this recommendation. Boards of Health and the selectmen of towns have ever had the management of these matters in this State. There are few if any states or countries, where more excellent regulations relating to the burial-grounds and the interment of the dead exist, where the ceremony of burial is conducted with more propriety, and where greater respect is paid to the deceased. Yet in some particulars improvement might and ought to be made. The history and condition of burial-grounds, and the regulations for the interment of the dead, are intimately connected with public health, and should form a part of the sanitary regulations of every city and town. . . .

XXXIV. We recommend *that measures be taken to preserve the lives and the health of passengers at sea, and of seamen engaged in the merchant service.*

Vessels at sea are the floating habitations of living beings; and in these, as in dwellings on the land, the air may be corrupted by over-crowding, filth, and other causes, and thus become a fruitful source of disease. "Of all known poisons," says Dr. [Andrew] Combe, "that produced by the concentrated effluvia from a crowd of human beings, confined within a small space, and neglectful of cleanliness, is one of the worst; and in ships where ventilation is not enforced,—especially if the passengers are dirty in their habits, and much kept below by bad weather,—it frequently operates with an intensity which no constitution can long resist." ...

Without attempting in this place to recommend a specific system of sanitary regulations for ships, we urge, in general terms, upon merchants, sea-faring men, and others interested, the great importance of the subject. Dryness, ventilation, and cleanliness, should be enforced in every department of the ship; foul and putrid cargoes should be avoided; and every means used, by proper diet and regimen, to preserve the health of the seamen and passengers. Sanitary improvement was early introduced on board ships, as we shall presently show; and a great number of human lives have consequently been saved. In no department of social economy can preventive measures have a greater influence. Boards of Health might do a good service to humanity, by issuing a simple and judicious code of sanitary regulations for ships.

XXXV. We recommend *that the authority to make regulations for the quarantine of vessels be instrusted to the local Boards of Health.*

The seventeenth section of the proposed act contains all necessary authority for making quarantine regulations. Boards of Health in sea-port towns will be able to obtain all needful information regarding their duties, by consulting the works referred to in the appendix, and making such regulations as are adapted to their own peculiar circumstances. The extremely valuable Report of the General Board of Health of England on Quarantine, published last year, is particularly commended. Public opinion on this subject seems to have undergone a great change within a few years past.

XXXVI. We recommend *that measures be adopted for preventing or mitigating the sanitary evils arising from foreign emigration.*

This recommendation involves one of the most momentous, profound, and difficult social problems ever presented to us for solution. . . .

We will not attempt to suggest a remedy for this most pregnant anomaly. It requires to be more carefully studied, and more thoroughly surveyed than the present occasion allows. The State should pass suitable laws on the subject, and the general and local Boards of Health should carefully observe these evils in all their sanitary bearings and relations. We would, however, suggest:

1. That emigration, especially of paupers, invalids, and criminals, should, by all proper means, be discouraged; and that misrepresentation and falsehood, to induce persons to embark in passenger-ships, should be discountenanced and counteracted.

2. That ship-owners and others should be held to strict accountability for all expenses of pauper emigrants, and that existing bonds for their support should be strictly enforced.

3. That a system be devised by which all emigrants, or those who introduce them, by water or by land, should be required to pay a sufficient sum to create a general sinking fund for the support of all who may require aid in the State, at least within five years after their arrival.

4. That such a description of each emigrant be registered as will afford the means of identification of any one, at any time, and in any place, within five or more years after arrival.

5. That encouragement be given to emigrate from places in this State, where there is little demand for labor, to other places; and that associations be formed among the emigrants for settling on the public lands of the United States.

6. That efforts be made, by all proper means, to elevate the sanitary and social condition of foreigners, and to promote among them habits of cleanliness and better modes of living.

7. That our system of social and personal charitable relief should be revised and remodeled, and that a general plan be devised which shall bring all the charities of the city, county and state, under one control, and thus prevent injudicious almsgiving and imposition.

8. That an establishment for paupers, including a farm and workshops, be formed in each county in the State, to which State paupers might be sent, and where they should be required to labor, as far as practicable, for their support.

Most of these recommendations may be carried into effect without any special legislative authority, State or municipal.

XXXVII. We recommend *that a sanitary association be formed in every city and town in the State, for the purpose of collecting and diffusing information relating to public and personal health.*

The subject of sanitary improvement is comparatively new. Few minds, in this country at least have as yet been led to examine it, to see its bearing upon the welfare and progress of humanity. Those, however, who have looked at it with any considerable degree of care, have been convinced of its importance; and it only requires to be generally understood to be universally regarded as *the* great subject of the age. Public opinion needs to be educated, and in no way can it be more effectually done than by associated effort. If a Metropolitan Sanitary Association existed in Boston, as a central agency, and a Branch Sanitary Association in every city and town in the State, they might do much to effect this object, by collecting and diffusing useful information; and, by their cooperation with the public authorities, render the discharge of their duties comparatively more easy. Inestimable benefits might thus be secured to the cause and to the people. To aid those who may wish to form such associations, we suggest the sub-joined form of a constitution. . .

City Public Health Departments Are Established

The New York City Department of Health and Mental Hygiene

In 1805 the city of New York established its first Board of Health to combat a yellow fever epidemic that was spreading throughout the northeastern seaboard. The epidemic struck in Philadelphia first and then appeared in New York in the late 1700s. It quickly became obvious to city leaders in New York that imposing quarantine alone was not enough to deal with the crisis and that sanitation rules had to be passed and enforced. Thus, the Board of Health was born.

The story of the evolution of New York City's Board of Health is the subject of the following article. Rules governing the sanitation of New York City took a long time to arrive, however. In its early days the Board of Health merely reacted to outbreaks of disease as best it could. As the article suggests, the members of the Board of Health often bowed to either the pressures of the political machines that ran the city or the business community that dared not stop the flow of commerce into and out of the metropolis. By the mid-1800s reformers began to call for the creation of a totally independent health department. In 1866, the Metropolitan Board of Health was established. For its time, the board was the most powerful public health body in the nation.

Yellow fever sparked the formation of New York's first Board of Health. In the summer of 1793, when an epidemic killed 5,000 in nearby Philadelphia, a group of leading doctors in New York organized a committee to prevent boats from Philadelphia from entering New York's ports. These quarantine efforts may have helped keep the disease away that

The New York City Department of Health and Mental Hygiene, "Protecting Public Health in New York City: 200 Years of Leadership." www.nyc.gov.

summer. But in the summers of 1795, 1799, and 1803, Yellow Fever, which caused victims to develop a yellowed complexion and vomit black bile, felled thousands of New Yorkers. These epidemics lent weight to the view that sanitary measures, and not just quarantine, were needed to curb the disease. The city's Common Council consequently determined that it needed greater authority over local sanitation to control Yellow Fever. So on January 17, 1805, it passed an ordinance to create the first New York City Board of Health, made up of Mayor De Witt Clinton and a committee of city aldermen.

Reacting to Crises

Over the next half-century, the Board generally took a reactive stance, meeting whenever an epidemic threatened the city. Between outbreaks of disease, city government paid little attention to health. While the Board spent more than $25,000 fighting Yellow Fever in 1805, its budget dropped to $1,500 the next year and funds did not increase until the city faced another epidemic in 1819. Between 1822, the last time Yellow Fever struck the city, and 1832, when Asiatic cholera reached New York for the first time, the board was inactive. In the 1840s, the board met rarely until cholera again struck the city in 1849. In these early years, public health became a political concern only when disease brought the bustling city to a standstill.

Even in times of dire crisis, the Board proved unpredictable. In 1805, its members acted swiftly when Yellow Fever cases appeared, ordering patients removed to the Marine Hospital on Staten Island, evacuating residents from sections of the city where the disease had struck, and appointing night watchmen to guard abandoned areas. The Board also erected a temporary asylum to house poor families that had been evacuated, and provided rations for families who were starving due to lack of work in the desolate city. Similarly, in the epidemic of 1819, "[i]mmediate measures were adopted to clear the sickly district of its inhabitants, and to fence up the avenues which led to the seat of infection," according to Mayor Stephen Allen. But in 1822, the last time a Yellow Fever epidemic struck New York, the Board hesitated to declare the disease present.

By the time the Board had shut affected areas, most residents, recognizing the disease from previous years, had packed up and moved to temporary homes, banks, and shops in nearby Greenwich Village, which was then a small town north of the city's limits.

After each epidemic, the City Inspector's office provided a detailed statistical account of mortality. John Pintard, a prominent merchant and former state assemblyman, began privately collecting mortality statistics for New York in 1802, and two years later, the city appointed him its first inspector to keep official mortality statistics. Pintard hoped that statistics would increase knowledge of disease among physicians and the general public. The November 1805 City Inspector's Report, he wrote, was designed to "furnish data for reflection and calculation," in order that the "awful malady" of Yellow Fever could one day "become more controllable and less mortal." That year, there had been 600 reported cases and 262 deaths from Yellow Fever. The city inspector's mortality statistics would prove invaluable in demonstrating the gravity of the city's health problems in the 1840s and 1850s.

The Concerns over Commerce

The arrival of Asiatic cholera stirred the Board to action as the Yellow Fever epidemics had earlier. Upon hearing that cholera was ravaging Europe in late 1831, the Board quarantined ships from Europe and enacted measures to clean the city's dirty streets. But once cholera cases began to appear in the city, the Board was slow to recognize them, as cholera would interrupt the flow of commerce. The Board was "more afraid of merchants than of lying," one prominent resident, William Dunlap, wrote to a friend that year. During the 1849 epidemic, the Board tried to act, but faced hostility from land-lords when it tried to set up a cholera hospital and had to use the second floor of a tavern and four public schools as a makeshift facility. The Board's Sanatory Committee managed to get the police to remove between five and six thousand hogs from crowded tenement areas—a measure thought to re-duce disease—even after residents rioted in protest. The Board and City Inspector's Office also shut the bone-boiling plants that disposed of animal carcasses. as these centrally-located businesses were considered a disease-causing nuisance. But this just meant that the carcasses were thrown into the river to rot near the docks.

As wealthier residents fled to the country during the chol-era epidemics, the disease was left to ravage the poor, mostly free blacks and Irish immigrants. Of the 5,017 who died dur-ing the 1849 epidemic, a full 40 percent had been born in Ire-land. While the city had absorbed just over 92,000 immigrants between 1820 and 1830, over 1.1 million arrived between 1840 and 1850, and 1.2 million between 1850 and 1860. Many middle-class Germans and other Europeans arrived in these years, but most immigrants were fleeing famine-starved Ire-land. The Irish soon occupied the increasingly crowded dis-tricts of New York centered on the Five Points neighborhood. Immigration fueled demand for housing and led unscrupu-lous landlords to erect tenements such as one on Mulberry Street that by 1849 had "800 persons crowded upon two lots, six persons living in almost every room." The squalor of tene-ments spilled onto the city streets: corrupt city officials awarded street cleaning contracts as political patronage, with little expectation that the jobs would get done. The streets were filled with rotting garbage, dead animals, and overflow-ing human and animal waste. Hogs, dogs, and other animals ran wild in the poorer neighborhoods. The city had little in-centive to curb the hog population, as these scavengers were the only effective street cleaners.

Clean Water

The 1832 cholera epidemic, which even then was known to be associated with dirty water, did spur one civic improvement. In the following years, the city's Common Council ordered water commissioners to draw up a plan for an aqueduct to bring clean water to the city, which voters later approved. The Croton Aqueduct and reservoir, which brought water from the Croton River to the city's pipe system, opened on October 14, 1842 at a cost of $11.5 million. The water was used for drinking and street cleaning, although the Croton Water Board objected, even during the 1849 cholera epidemic, to using the water to clean streets in the Five Points area.

While the city's wealthier Protestant classes generally blamed the cholera epidemics on supposed moral failures of the Irish—Catholicism, drinking, and poverty—some reform-minded citizens began to see crowded tenement housing as the root of the problem. The Association for Improving the Condition of the Poor, an organization founded in 1843, began campaigning to improve these conditions. Physician-reformers, including Dr. Elisha Harris and Dr. John Griscom, also called for landlords to erect healthy tenements with better ventilation and more space. But tenement conditions and the health of their residents only worsened during the decade. By 1863, the death rate in the tenement-filled Sixth Ward was triple that of the city overall with infant mortality as a leading cause of death. By 1860, many more people were dying every year than were being born: In a population of over 814,000, there were almost twice as many deaths (22,710) as births (12,454).

Calls for Reform

In the late 1850s, reformers began calling for the state legislature to establish an independent city health department that would not be controlled by the corrupt Tammany machine [Democratic Party political machine that controlled New York

City politics for decades]. The first public health bill proposing such a department was introduced in 1859. The draft riots of 1863, in which Irish immigrants attacked black residents and more than 1,000 people died, caused many wealthy citizens to sign on to the reformers' cause, as they saw that tenement conditions could produce mass violence. A new group, the Citizens' Association, drew together prominent residents including Peter Cooper and Hamilton Fish, and physician-reformers such as John Griscom, Elisha Harris, Willard Parker, Stephen Smith, and James Wood. But it would take six failed health bills and the threat of a new cholera epidemic before the Association's efforts succeeded. On February 26, 1866, amid reports that cholera was again headed to New York, the state legislature passed a new public health law that created the Metropolitan Board of Health. The new Board encompassed Kings, Richmond, Westchester, part of Queens, and New York counties. Under the law, the Board included a president, four police commissioners, a health officer, and four other commissioners appointed by the Governor. Importantly, at least three of these commissioners had to be physicians. Health in the city no longer lay under the sole control of politicians.

The new Board, led by the energetic Jackson Schultz, hired a phalanx of sanitary inspectors to curb cholera. When a case was reported, a crew was dispatched to disinfect the home of the victim and remove soiled garments. This corps of inspectors acted on new scientific evidence that cholera was transmitted through the excreta and bedclothes of the victims. The Board also sought to provide food and clothing for families of cholera victims. Partly due to these efforts, New York suffered a tenth the number of cholera deaths in 1866 that it had in 1849. This triumph showed how the Board—which under the new law had been rendered more powerful than any other local public health body in the United States—could stem the tide of epidemic disease.

Cleaning up the city proved a more difficult task. In 1866, the Board ordered 160,000 tons of manure removed from vacant lots, 4,000 yards to be cleaned, and 6,418 privies to be disinfected. The Board "coerced and stimulated the public schools and other institutional authorities of the district to regard sanitary laws," pressured landlords to clean up their buildings, and sought to suppress "cattle-driving in the day time" and to control animal slaughtering. In 1869, the Board resolved that "neither hogs nor goats could run at large in our city within its jurisdiction, neither could they be kept within 1,000 feet of any residence or business without a permit from the Board of Health."

Return to Political Control

By 1870, the Board's brief honeymoon seemed to be ending. "Boss" William Tweed, head of Tammany Hall, provided the city with a new charter, returning control over health matters to the city. He created a new Health Department with a Board of Health to oversee it. While similar in composition to the previous Metropolitan Board of Health, this Board included members appointed by the Mayor rather than the Governor. The Department was organized into four bureaus: a Bureau of Sanitary Inspection, a Bureau of Records and Inspection, a Bureau of Street Cleaning, and a Bureau of Sanitary Permits. Even when the Department and Board were headed by corrupt Tammany Hall appointees, the physicians, and other experts in these divisions created a buttress against political influence.

Charles F. Chandler, a professor of chemistry at Columbia University, exemplified the new scientific character of the Health Department. Beginning in the late 1860s, he directed a Department chemical laboratory that examined water, milk, and food supplies. Chandler, who was named Health Commissioner in 1873, worked for more than a decade to sanitize the city within the constraints of an inadequate budget. He appointed the city's first milk inspector, but had a staff of only 14 health inspectors, sharply limiting the Department's impact.

Teaching the Public About Health and Hygiene

Karen Buhler-Wilkerson

The improvement of sanitation and hygiene was the mandate of the nation's earliest boards of health. In the 1800s and early 1900s municipalities throughout the nation built massive public works projects such as sewer systems and waterworks to serve the rapidly growing urban centers. Yet one of the most daunting tasks was to teach city dwellers, many of them poor immigrants, about the importance of hygiene in improving health. The need to help the sick and educate people about hygiene is the topic of the selection that follows.

As described by author Karen Buhler-Wilkerson public health nursing in New York City began in the late 1800s with the establishment of the Visiting Nurse Service of New York (VNSNY). The VNSNY's mission was twofold: to help the poor and infirm of New York City and also alleviate the causes of disease through education and improved public health standards. What made the early visiting nurses unique was their commitment to living in the neighborhood with their clients and the broad view they took of the concept of "health." As envisioned by founders Lillian Wald and Mary Brewster, nurses had to attend to all aspects of the community in order to succeed in bringing about drastic change. Today's visiting nurses continue to work in the fields of home-health care and wherever they are needed.

A century ago, American cities were dirty, crowded, and unhealthy places to live. The fluctuating, dramatic, and often frightening presence of infectious disease was a source of great public concern. As popular knowledge of the germ

Karen Buhler-Wilkerson, "The Call to the Nurse: Our History from 1893 to 1943," *vnsny.org*, February 19, 2007. Reprinted by permission of Visiting Nurse Service of New York.

theory of disease spread, urban dwellers began to realize that individual health depended to some extent on the health of the general population. Not only was illness a major cause of destitution, but the infectious diseases contracted by poor people appeared to threaten the well-being of the middle and upper classes as well.

In response to these circumstances, hundreds of community organizations hired trained nurses to care for the sick poor in their homes. The image of the nurse climbing tenement stairs to save the poor from illness struck the fancy of many groups interested in social reform. By the turn of the century, women's clubs, churches, mission societies, hospitals, charity organizations, health departments, settlement houses, and tuberculosis and visiting nurse associations were hiring nurses to care for the sick. In so doing, the members of each group believed they were protecting the public from the spread of infectious disease. Such diversity of private and public sponsorship reflected both upper-class fear of diseases associated with the "dangerous classes" and recognition of the trained nurse as an economical and practical solution to the complex problem of "elevating" poor, often immigrant, families to a more ordered, healthier existence.

Henry Street Nurses Settlement, a visionary experiment, was founded in these socially turbulent times by Lillian Wald. Author of the term *public health nursing*, Wald was instrumental in securing reforms in health, industry, education, recreation, and housing. Her original ideas led to the establishment of the Federal Children's Bureau, school nursing, insurance payments for home-based nursing care, and a national public health nursing service.

Lillian Wald

This story begins in the late winter of 1893, when Wald learned that a Sabbath school for Immigrants needed a course in home nursing. Unaware of the work of those who had preceded her to New York's Lower East Side and even more ignorant of life's realities for most immigrants, Wald agreed to establish and teach the class. A call for help to the home of one of her immigrant students, Mrs. Lipsky, changed the course of nursing history within an hour. Wald later wrote of being guided by Mrs. Lipsky's young daughter, through crowded "evil-smelling" streets, past open courtyard "closets," up the slimy steps of a rear tenement, and finally into the sickroom:

> *All the maladjustments of our social and economic relations seemed epitomized in this brief journey and what was found at the end of it. The family to which the child led me was neither criminal nor vicious. Although the husband was a cripple, one of those who stand on street corners exhibiting deformities to enlist compassion, and masking the begging of alms by a pretense at selling; although the family of seven shared their rooms with boarders . . . and although the sick woman lay on a wretched, unclean bed, soiled with a hemorrhage two days old, they were not degraded human beings, judged by any measure of moral values. In fact, it was very plain that they were sensitive to their condition, and when, at the end of my ministrations, they kissed my hands . . . it would have been solace if by any conviction of the moral unworthiness of the family I could have defended myself as a part of a society which permitted such conditions to exist. Indeed, my subsequent acquaintance with them revealed the fact that, miserable as their state was, they were not without ideals for the family life, and for society, of which they were so unloved and unlovely a part.*

This experience for Wald was a baptism by fire. Naively convinced that such conditions existed only because "people did not know," Wald committed herself "to know and to tell." Rejoicing that her training in the care of the sick gave her an "organic relationship" to the community, she and Mary Brewster devised a plan to live in the neighborhood as nurses. . . .

Living in the Neighborhood

Free from any form of external control or regulation, Wald and Brewster moved to the Lower East Side in July of 1893, ". . . to do what they could; to see what they could see; and to publicize all that was wrong and remediable. . . ." They arrived at the moment of the country's worst depression. Confronted by the disease, poverty, and the filth of crowded tenement homes, Wald and Brewster immediately recognized that the sickness encountered had to be seen within the context of its social and economic impact on families. They always began by caring for the patient—putting him or her "in nursing condition" and arranging for someone to watch after the patient until the next nursing visit. Recovery, however, required much more than good nursing care.

By the end of a month on the Lower East Side, Wald began to mobilize a vast array of disjointed services to remedy her neighbors' ills, from private relief agencies to the medical establishment itself. Creation of cooperative relationships with organizations as varied as newspapers and hospitals allowed Wald to provide patients with ice, sterilized milk, medicines, and meals. As word of the nurses' work spread, hospitals, dispensaries, relief agencies, and private physicians became "believers," referring neighborhood patients for skilled care, follow-up, and teaching. . . .

Using the authority given them by the Board of Health, Wald and Brewster began a neighborhood campaign to clean roofs, disinfect "vaults," and clean up tenement hallways, while "greater nuisances" (offensive stables) were referred to the Board of Health in their daily reports. Wald and Brewster, willingly washed dirt from their patients, claiming "the use of scrubbing brush and bath has been frequent—if we can't assert it to be permanent." Any real household or personal "transformations" were rewarded with new clothes or linens. . . .

"Community Mother"

Anxious for neighborhood residents to experience a life other than that associated with crowded tenement and factory, Wald regularly arranged for amenities and social pleasures, everything from flowers to country excursions, picnics, and concert tickets. Mothers were coaxed to send their children to school (sometimes with the aid of a truant officer) and "little bank accounts" were opened in children's names to save any extra money earned. During the nurses' first holiday season, neighbors reciprocated, coming to "sing to us and some brought . . . little cards, passed most apparently through more hands than one. . . ."

By providing care for their neighbors' numerous illnesses, assisting in death and "alas many births," as well as making countless visits "for other purposes . . . as varied as the people," Wald became for the Lower East Side and the country, the first public health nurse. She was what public health leader C.E.A. Winslow would later dub a "community mother"—the trained and scientific representative of the good neighbor, caring for all, sick and well.

Wald chose the term "public health nurse" to emphasize the "community value of the nurse" and the relationship of public health nursing to the social problems that invariably accompany a patient's individual illness. Whether problems were isolated and peculiar, or common to many was, according to Wald, important to determine because the "technique for finding out" often led logically to identification of the remedy. From the beginning, every incident that "seemed to have community bearing" was noted and held in reserve for such time as it could be "broadcast to enable others with facilities for greater publicity to influence and educate public opinion toward pricked consciences and mutual responsibility."

The Settlement as Local Hospital and School

By Passover of 1895, Wald reported that their neighbors still visited, choosing to take "tea with us as their celebration." She concluded, "We are not tired of them nor they, apparently, of us." The continued welcome, notwithstanding, Wald's desire to create a larger, more formal organization made it necessary to move from the tenement to a nearby house which would become the Henry Street Nurses Settlement. At the May meeting of the National Conference of Charities and Corrections, Wald solicited "zealous women" of talent, personality, ability, and spirit to realize the privilege of joining the "family." She hoped to limit the settlement's members to six nurses representing the training and connections of a variety of nursing schools, and bringing an esprit de corps essential to cooperative work. The settlement nurses would receive a "fellowship," but would share collectively in living expenses.

One room of the settlement was reserved as a dispensary where simple nursing cases could be treated and where physicians could attend to special cases not requiring treatment in the larger clinics scattered throughout the city. An extra bathroom was set aside for regular and emergency use, particularly to prepare neighbors for trips to the country in summer. Finally, classes in home nursing, making of poultices, care of bed patients, elementary first aid to the injured, household hygiene, and child care were conducted for mothers and children from the tenements. . . .

Nurses from Henry Street Settlement were available throughout the city seven days a week between the hours of 8:30 a.m. and 5 p.m. Patients were usually visited on a daily basis and night nurses, along with cleaning and laundry services, were provided for the critically ill. As a rule, new cases were seen first, morning and afternoon. Patients with elevated temperatures or in poor condition were usually seen twice a day, often with the second visit to make them comfortable for the night. . . .

In 1933, after 40 years on the Lower East Side, Lillian Wald retired as head of Henry Street Settlement. By now, her staff of 265 annually climbed 24,750 tenement stairs, drove 140,000 miles and took 120,000 subway rides to make 550,000 home visits to 100,000 patients. The nurses cared for one-fourth of the cases of pneumonia, one-third of the maternity patients, and one-fifth of the "reportable" diseases in the city. . . .

Lillian Wald died in 1940 at her home in Westport, Connecticut, after a long illness. In 1944, social services and nursing activities were separated into distinct entities. The nursing service moved its headquarters farther uptown, becoming Visiting Nurse Service of New York, while Henry Street Settlement has remained focused on the neighborhoods of the Lower East Side.

An Exposé About Meatpacking Gives Birth to the Food and Drug Act

Upton Sinclair

The publication of The Jungle *by Upton Sinclair in 1906 exposed the unsanitary conditions of the nation's meatpacking industry and the harrowing work conditions of the meat packers. The descriptions of the slaughter of livestock and the processing of the meat described in the following passages galvanized the public and government and led to the establishment of the Pure Food and Drug Act and the Meat Inspection Act of 1906.*

The 1906 law protected the health of the public by prohibiting interstate and foreign commerce in adulterated and misbranded food and drugs. Drugs had to meet standards of purity and quality established by committees of physicians and pharmacists and food producers could not remove certain ingredients, substitute one ingredient for another, or add harmful ingredients to reduce the quality of their product. In addition, producers could not sell spoiled meat or vegetables. Misbranding of any food or drug was also prohibited. As described by Sinclair, the least desirable cuts of meat or spoiled meat were packaged and sold to the unsuspecting buyer as first quality.

The Bureau of Chemistry enforced the 1906 law until 1927 when it was reorganized. The Food, Drug, and Insecticide Administration was formed and renamed the Food and Drug Administration (FDA) in 1931. Two decades later the FDA became part of the Department of Health, Education, and Welfare—today the Department of Health and Human Services.

They passed down the busy street that led to the yards [Lithuanian immigrants Jurgis and Elzbieta are given a tour of the cattle yards by another immigrant]. It was still

Upton Sinclair, *The Jungle*, 1906. sunsite.berkeley.edu.

early morning, and everything was at its high tide of activity. A steady stream of employees was pouring through the gate—employees of the higher sort, at this hour, clerks and stenographers and such. For the women there were waiting big two-horse wagons, which set off at a gallop as fast as they were filled. In the distance there was heard again the lowing of the cattle, a sound as of a far-off ocean calling. They followed it, this time, as eager as children in sight of a circus menagerie—which, indeed, the scene a good deal resembled. They crossed the railroad tracks, and then on each side of the street were the pens full of cattle; they would have stopped to look, but Jokubas hurried them on, to where there was a stairway and a raised gallery, from which everything could be seen. Here they stood, staring, breathless with wonder.

There is over a square mile of space in the yards, and more than half of it is occupied by cattle pens; north and south as far as the eye can reach there stretches a sea of pens. And they were all filled—so many cattle no one had ever dreamed existed in the world. Red cattle, black, white, and yellow cattle; old cattle and young cattle; great bellowing bulls and little calves not an hour born; meek-eyed milch [milk] cows and fierce, long-horned Texas steers. The sound of them here was as of all the barnyards of the universe; and as for counting them—it would have taken all day simply to count the pens. . . .

"And what will become of all these creatures?" cried Teta Elzbieta.

"By tonight," Jokubas answered, "they will all be killed and cut up; and over there on the other side of the packing houses are more railroad tracks, where the cars come to take them away."

Creatures Turned into Food

There were two hundred and fifty miles of track within the yards, their guide went on to tell them. They brought about ten thousand head of cattle every day, and as many hogs, and half as many sheep—which meant some eight or ten million live creatures turned into food every year. One stood and watched, and little by little caught the drift of the tide, as it set in the direction of the packing houses. There were groups of cattle being driven to the chutes, which were roadways about fifteen feet wide, raised high above the pens. In these chutes the stream of animals was continuous; it was quite uncanny to watch them, pressing on to their fate, all unsuspicious a very river of death. Our friends were not poetical, and the sight suggested to them no metaphors of human destiny; they thought only of the wonderful efficiency of it all. The chutes into which the hogs went climbed high up—to the very top of the distant buildings; and Jokubas explained that the hogs went up by the power of their own legs, and then their weight carried them back through all the processes necessary to make them into pork.

"They don't waste anything here," said the guide, and then he laughed and added a witticism, which he was pleased that his unsophisticated friends should take to be his own: "They use everything about the hog except the squeal." In front of Brown's General Office building there grows a tiny plot of grass, and this, you may learn, is the only bit of green thing in Packingtown; likewise this jest about the hog and his squeal, the stock in trade of all the guides, is the one gleam of humor that you will find there. . . .

Inside the Slaughterhouse

It was a long, narrow room, with a gallery along it for visitors. At the head there was a great iron wheel, about twenty feet in circumference, with rings here and there along its edge. Upon both sides of this wheel there was a narrow space, into which came the hogs at the end of their journey; in the midst of them stood a great burly Negro, bare-armed and bare-chested. He was resting for the moment, for the wheel had stopped while men were cleaning up. In a minute or two, however, it began slowly to revolve, and then the men upon each side of it sprang to work. They had chains which they fastened about the leg of the nearest hog, and the other end of the chain they hooked into one of the rings upon the wheel. So, as the wheel turned, a hog was suddenly jerked off his feet and borne aloft.

At the same instant the car was assailed by a most terrifying shriek; the visitors started in alarm, the women turned pale and shrank back. The shriek was followed by another, louder and yet more agonizing—for once started upon that journey, the hog never came back; at the top of the wheel he was shunted off upon a trolley, and went sailing down the room. And meantime another was swung up, and then another, and another, until there was a double line of them, each dangling by a foot and kicking in frenzy—and squealing. The uproar was appalling, perilous to the eardrums; one feared there was too much sound for the room to hold—that the walls must give way or the ceiling crack. There were high squeals and low squeals, grunts, and wails of agony; there would come a momentary lull, and then a fresh outburst, louder than ever, surging up to a deafening climax. It was too much for some of the visitors—the men would look at each other, laughing nervously, and the women would stand with hands clenched, and the blood rushing to their faces, and the tears starting in their eyes.

Meantime, heedless of all these things, the men upon the floor were going about their work. Neither squeals of hogs nor tears of visitors made any difference to them; one by one they hooked up the hogs, and one by one with a swift stroke they slit their throats. There was a long line of hogs, with squeals and lifeblood ebbing away together; until at last each started again, and vanished with a splash into a huge vat of boiling water.

It was all so very businesslike that one watched it fascinated. It was porkmaking by machinery, porkmaking by applied mathematics....

The Immigrant Family Working in the Processing Plants

With one member trimming beef in a cannery, and another working in a sausage factory, the family had a first-hand knowledge of the great majority of Packingtown swindles. For it was the custom, as they found, whenever meat was so spoiled that it could not be used for anything else, either to can it or else to chop it up into sausage. With what had been told them by Jonas, who had worked in the pickle rooms, they could now study the whole of the spoiled-meat industry on the inside, and read a new and grim meaning into that old Packingtown jest—that they use everything of the pig except the squeal.

Jonas had told them how the meat that was taken out of pickle would often be found sour, and how they would rub it up with soda to take away the smell, and sell it to be eaten on free-lunch counters; also of all the miracles of chemistry which they performed, giving to any sort of meat, fresh or salted, whole or chopped, any color and any flavor and any odor they chose. In the pickling of hams they had an ingenious apparatus, by which they saved time and increased the capacity of the plant—a machine consisting of a hollow needle attached to a pump; by plunging this needle into the meat and working with his foot, a man could fill a ham with pickle in a few seconds. And yet, in spite of this, there would be hams found spoiled, some of them with an odor so bad that a man could hardly bear to be in the room with them. To pump into these the packers had a second and much stronger pickle which destroyed the odor—a process known to the workers as "giving them thirty per cent." Also, after the hams had been smoked, there would be found some that had gone to the bad. Formerly these had been sold as "Number Three Grade," but later on some ingenious person had hit upon a new device, and now they would extract the bone, about which the bad part generally lay, and insert in the hole a white-hot iron. After this invention there was no longer Number One, Two, and Three Grade—there was only Number One Grade. The packers were always originating such schemes—they had what they called "boneless hams," which were all the odds and ends of pork stuffed into casings; and "California hams," which were the shoulders, with big knuckle joints, and nearly all the meat cut out; and fancy "skinned hams," which were made of the oldest hogs, whose skins were so heavy and coarse that no one would buy them—that is, until they had been cooked and chopped fine and labeled "head cheese!"

It was only when the whole ham was spoiled that it came into the department of Elzbieta. Cut up by the two-thousand-revolutions-a-minute flyers, and mixed with half a ton of other meat, no odor that ever was in a ham could make any difference. There was never the least attention paid to what was cut up for sausage; there would come all the way back from Europe old sausage that had been rejected, and that was moldy and white—it would be dosed with borax and glycerine, and dumped into the hoppers, and made over again for home consumption. There would be meat that had tumbled out on the floor, in the dirt and sawdust, where the workers had tramped and spit uncounted billions of consumption germs. There would be meat stored in great piles in rooms; and the water from leaky roofs would drip over it, and thousands of rats would race about on it. It was too dark in these storage places to see well, but a man could run his hand over these piles of meat and sweep off handfuls of the dried dung of rats. These rats were nuisances, and the packers would put poisoned bread out for them; they would die, and then rats, bread, and meat would go into the hoppers together. This is no fairy story and no joke; the meat would be shoveled into carts, and the man who did the shoveling would not trouble to lift out a rat even when he saw one—there were things that went into the sausage in comparison with which a poisoned rat was a tidbit. There was no place for the men to wash their hands before they ate their dinner, and so they made a practice of washing them in the water that was to be ladled into the sausage. There were the butt-ends of smoked meat, and the scraps of corned beef, and all the odds and ends of the waste of the plants, that would be dumped into old barrels in the cellar and left there. Under the system of rigid economy which the packers enforced, there were some jobs that it only paid to do once in a long time, and among these was the cleaning out of the waste barrels. Every spring they did it; and in the barrels would be dirt and rust and old nails and stale water—and cartload after cartload of it would be taken up and dumped into the hoppers with fresh meat, and sent out to the public's breakfast. Some of it they would make into "smoked" sausage—but as the smoking took time, and was therefore expensive, they would call upon their chemistry department, and preserve it with borax and color it with gelatine to make it brown. All of their sausage came out of the same bowl, but when they came to wrap it they would stamp some of it "special," and for this they would charge two cents more a pound.

The Need to Protect the Public Health versus the Rights of the Individual

Mary Mallon

During the late 1800s and early 1900s scientists were trying to find cures for common diseases such as typhoid, cholera, tuberculosis, diphtheria, and others that were responsible for the deaths of hundreds of Americans each year. Lacking cures, the only weapon available to public health officials was quarantine, or the isolation of the infected persons or neighborhoods from the rest of the population. Quarantine was feared by many because of the stigma attached to the sick person and the loss of income from being separated from one's work. Quarantine also had legal ramifications. Did public health departments that enforced quarantine violate the sick person's rights? Or did the health and welfare of the larger public supersede those of the individual?

These questions arose during the dramatic case of Mary Mallon, an Irish immigrant cook who, although healthy, infected forty-seven people with typhoid fever. Mallon was hunted down by the authorities and quarantined on a small island in the middle of New York City's East River. Mallon was a poor, single woman who wanted to work at her trade but the city forbade her to do so. Mary Mallon wrote the following letter in 1909 from her place of quarantine. In it she protests her treatment. The next year the health commissioner took pity on Mallon and released her from quarantine under the provision that she not return to cooking. Despite the warning, Mallon resumed her old job and the outbreaks of typhoid appeared again. Mallon was arrested and placed in quarantine, this time for the rest of her life.

Mary Mallon, "To the Editor of the American," 1909. www.pbs.org/wgbh/nova.

In reply to Dr. Park of the Board of Health I will state that I am not segregated with the typhoid patients. There is nobody on this island that has typhoid. There was never any effort by the Board authority to do anything for me excepting to cast me on the island and keep me a prisoner without being sick nor needing medical treatment. When I first came here they took two blood cultures, and feces went down three times per week, say Monday, Wednesday, and Friday, respectively, until the latter part of June. After that they only got the feces once a week, which was on Wednesday. Now they have given me a record for nearly a year for three times a week.

When I first came here I was so nervous and almost prostrated with grief and trouble. My eyes began to twitch, and the left eyelid became paralyzed and would not move. It remained in that condition for six months. There was an eye specialist [who] visited the island three and four times a week. He was never asked to visit me. I did not even get a cover for my eye. I had to hold my hand on it whilst going about and at night tie a bandage on it.

In December when Dr. Wilson took charge, he came to me and I told him about it. He said that was news to him and that he would send me his electric battery, *but he never sent* [it]. However, my eye got better thanks to the *Almighty God* and . . . in spite of the medical staff. Dr. Wilson ordered me *urotropin*. I got that on and off for a year. Sometimes they had it, and sometimes they did not. I took the urotropin for about three months all told during the whole *year*. If I should have continued [it], it would certainly have killed me for it was very severe. Everyone knows who is acquainted in any kind of medicine that it's used for *kidney* trouble.

When in January [1908] they were about to discharge me, when the resident physician came to me and asked me where was I going when I got out of here, naturally I said to N.Y., so there was a stop put to my getting out of here. Then the supervising nurse told me I was a hopeless case, and if I'd write to Dr. Darlington and tell him I'd go to my sisters in Connecticut. Now I have no sister in that state or any other in the U.S. Then in April a friend of mine went to Dr. Darlington and asked him when I was to get away. He replied "That woman is all right now, and she is a very expensive woman, but I cannot let her go myself. The Board has to sit. Come around Saturday." When he did, Dr. Darlington told this man "I've nothing more to do with this woman. Go to Dr. Studdiford"

He went to that doctor, and he said "I cannot let that woman go, and all the people that she gave the typhoid to and so many deaths occurred in the families she was with." Dr. Studdiford said to this man "Go and ask Mary Mallon and enveigle [entice] her to have an operation performed to have her gallbladder removed. I'll have the best surgeon in town to do the cutting." I said "No. No knife will be put on me. I've nothing the matter with my gallbladder." Dr. Wilson asked me the very same question. I also told him no. Then he replied "It might not do you any good." Also the supervising nurse asked me to have an operation performed. I also told her no, and she made the remark "Would it not be better for you to have it done than remain here?" I told her no.

There is a visiting doctor who came here in October. He did take quite an interest in me. He really thought I liked it here, that I did not care for my freedom. He asked me if I'd take some medicine if he brought it to me. I said I would, so he brought me some Anti Autotox and some pills then. Dr. Wilson had already ordered me brewer's yeast. At first I would not take it, for I'm a little afraid of the people, and I have a good right for when I came to the Department they said they were in my [intestinal] tract. Later another said they were in the muscles of my bowels. And latterly they thought of the gallbladder.

I have been in fact a peep show for everybody. Even the interns had to come to see me and ask about the facts already known to the whole wide world. The tuberculosis men would say "There she is, the kidnapped woman." Dr. Park has had me illustrated in Chicago. I wonder how the said Dr. William H. Park would like to be insulted and put in the Journal and call him or his wife Typhoid William Park.

The Influenza Epidemic of 1918–1919 Shows Flaws in America's Public Health System

Alfred W. Crosby

Beginning in 1918 during World War I, and continuing into 1919, influenza spread throughout the world and the United States in one of the most severe outbreaks of infectious disease in the history of mankind. Named the "Spanish flu" from an outbreak in Spain in 1918 that killed 8 million in one month, the influenza circled the globe in weeks and months killing between 20 and 40 million people, more than were killed in the war. Scholars still debate where the flu first appeared but it most likely was spread by soldiers being transported around the globe on ships, trains, and other means of transport. People infected with the disease died within hours of infection. Young adults were particularly vulnerable.

In the following excerpt, historian Alfred W. Crosby describes how the Spanish flu swept the United States. He notes how the flu first appeared among soldiers and sailors and then leapt from region to region, afflicting some and bypassing others. At first, officials underplayed the outbreak of the flu and did little to respond to the fatalities. The focus of the nation was on winning the war for the Allies not on what seemed to be just an outbreak of a bad cold strain. Physicians lacked today's advanced bacteriological tests and misdiagnosed the flu as pneumonia. Finally, the United States did not have an efficient network of federal, state, and local public health departments to gather data on the disease or even provide a sketch of the epidemic.

Alfred W. Crosby, *America's Forgotten Pandemic: The Influenza of 1918*. New York: Cambridge University Press, 2003. © Alfred W. Crosby 2003. © Cambridge University Press 1989. Reprinted with the permission of Cambridge University Press.

The pandemic in the United States is succinctly described in three sets of figures: the numbers of flu and pneumonia deaths, week by week, of the three great categories of Americans in 1918: sailors, soldiers, and civilians. It might be better to use the statistics on cases, rather than deaths, as our measure, but influenza wasn't made a reportable disease for civilians in most parts of the nation until after the pandemic was in full flame, and even after that the case statistics were collected and sent to the Census Bureau from areas where only 77.8 percent of the estimated civilian population lived. The best weekly mortality statistics we have are for 45 of the nation's largest cities. The rises and declines of these latter statistics probably preceded those of the entire population by several days and more, because the pandemic penetrated and then departed from the rural areas later than the cities: but these numbers are good enough for our purpose, if their limitations are kept in mind. . . .

The Navy's Role in Spreading the Disease

Spanish influenza reached a peak first among navy personnel on shore duty in the United States in the last week of September, just as the federal government bestirred itself to do something about the pandemic. The reasons for the navy's being first were, of course, that the new wave had started in the navy and also that navy shore personnel were concentrated on the coast nearest the war, where the wave had its initial American focus. (Sailors at sea and overseas were another matter.) Soldiers and civilians, in contrast, were dispersed all over the continent, many in localities which remained free of disease for weeks after the Commonwealth Pier [in Boston] outbreak.

In fact, in the pandemic's first weeks it was largely a naval affair. The navy reduced travel between stations "to a minimum consistent with the requirements of war," but sailors or "Jackies," as the newspapers called them, did yeoman service in carrying Spanish influenza to all parts of the nation. On

September 7 a draft of Jackies from Boston arrived at the Philadelphia Naval Yard, where six cases of flu appeared on the eleventh. A draft of hundreds of men left that Naval Yard September 10 and six cases developed among them upon their arrival in Quebec the next day. On September 17 another draft of hundreds from the Philadelphia Naval Yard arrived at the Puget Sound Naval Yard in the state of Washington. Eleven were ill with flu on arrival, and the disease became epidemic in Seattle about September 25.

The navy's role in spreading the disease was not restricted to seaports. Special navy training detachments existed at colleges across the nation, and there was one very large naval base a thousand miles from the Atlantic: the Great Lakes Training Station thirty-odd miles north of Chicago. Flu first appeared at this station on September 11, and in a week there were 2,600 in a hospital prepared for no more than 1,800. All liberty for men of the Great Lakes Station was canceled on September 19, but it was much too late. The pandemic started in Chicago, the nation's biggest rail center, about three days later, moving from the northern suburbs, nearest the naval station, to the south.

The pandemic among army personnel in the United States didn't crest until the week ending October 11, two weeks later than it peaked among navy personnel. There were many more doughboys [soldiers] than Jackies, and the majority of them were in the interior, not on the coasts. However, these factors meant that the soldier, while often not the first to bring flu, did so in many more counties, villages, and towns than did the sailor. Time and again, the first news of local influenza in a city's newspapers referred to army camps and army personnel. The first flu appeared in Kentucky about September 27 when troops coming through from Texas on the Louisville and Nashville Railroad stopped off in Bowling Green, infected a few of the citizenry, got back on the train, and went on their way. Flu was brought to southern Illinois, specifically to Elco, a village of 236, by a soldier home on leave from Camp Forest, Georgia, with "a cold." He infected his fiancée, his cousin, and the postmaster's daughter, and in the next few days nearly every household in town had at least one case. Then he went back to take up the defense of democracy.

Rapid spread of any respiratory disease among army travelers was guaranteed by the army policy of taking fullest advantage of the space available to transport troops. In the day-coaches of troop trains three men squashed into every double seat, and on the sleepers one man slept in the upper berth and two in the lower. The miserable fate of the 239 men of the 328th Labor Battalion is an extreme example of what could happen under such conditions. The 328th boarded the train in Louisiana at 4:00 P.M. on September 26 with twelve men already sick, and arrived at Newport News, Virginia, for overseas shipment at 2:00 P.M. on the twenty-ninth. One hundred and twenty men developed influenza en route, and 61 more within a day or two after reaching Virginia. When the trip started, the 328th was an asset: when it ended, the 328th was a liability.

Slowing down the whole war machine was less dangerous than trying to hold it at top speed during the pandemic. Troop shipments to France were cut by 10 percent and more, the number of soldiers for each seat and berth on troop trains was reduced to one, and on October 11 the War Department ordered a reduction in the intensity of training at all army camps. At the end of the month, the Chief of Staff in Washington wired General [John J.] Pershing that the flu had stopped nearly all draft calls and practically all training in October.

Civilians Fall Ill

The pandemic reached its peak among American civilians two weeks or more after it crested for the army. A large proportion of the civilian population was not of ages especially susceptible to Spanish influenza, civilians were not crammed into camps where a sneeze was always a communal event, nor were civilians shunted about the country in large numbers in spite of incipient malaise.

But, of course, civilians engaged in long-range transportation could transmit flu with an efficiency almost equal to that of the military. Five days after the first cases appeared at Commonwealth Pier, the steamship *Harold Walker* cleared Boston for Tampico, Mexico, and New Orleans, arriving at the Louisiana port two weeks later. Fifteen of her crew had flu on the voyage and three died. The first cases of the newest and most virulent strain of Spanish influenza in both Tampico and New Orleans were almost certainly off the *Harold Walker*. Merchant seamen and railroad men must have been the vanguard of the pandemic in hundreds of cities and towns. . . .

Neither the United States Navy, the United States Army, nor the United States of America went through the pandemic as monolithic units. The pandemic lasted for months, and the sailors at Commonwealth Pier were done with the worst of it before their fellow Jackies in San Francisco caught their first dose of it. Boston and, for that matter, Seattle passed the peak of their epidemics weeks before the disease even reached the San Juan Islands in Puget Sound.

Spanish influenza moved across the United States in the same way as the pioneers had, for it followed their trails, which had become railroads, and propagated fastest in those localities most attractive to them—the confluences of rivers and trails, the easiest mountain passes, and the shortest portages, where they and their descendants had built their cities. The pandemic started along the axis from Massachusetts to Virginia where the pioneers had started, bypassed backwaters like northern Maine, leaped the Appalachians, and touched down at points, many of which the Indians, French, and English had known in their time and valued for their strategic positions along the inland waterways: Buffalo, Cleveland, Detroit, and Chicago on the Great Lakes system and Minneapolis, Louisville, Little Rock [Arkansas], Greenville [Mississippi] and New Orleans on the Mississippi system. At the same time, as if as anxious for westing as the Forty-niners, it jumped clear across the plains and the Rockies to Los Angeles, San Francisco, and Seattle. Then, with secure bases on both coasts and a grip on the chief interior lines of commerce, Spanish influenza, again like the pioneers, took its time to seep into every niche and corner of America.

But this description implies more uniformity than really existed. Why did the pandemic, which reached Philadelphia and Pittsburgh at approximately the same time, crest in the former in the third week of October, but not till three weeks later in the latter? Why did New York City, one of the earliest cities to be infected, have a lower death rate than any other major city in the East? Why should the death rate in Chicago have been three times that of Grand Rapids, Michigan, less than 200 miles away and closely tied to Chicago by several transportation systems? Why did two towns, Darien and Milford, in Connecticut, a small and heavily infected state, crisscrossed by roads and railroads, escape the mortality of Spanish influenza completely?

Why were some areas and cities visited by severe return waves of the disease, such as Louisville, Kentucky, which suffered three crests—October and December 1918, and March 1919—while others, like Philadelphia and Albany [New York], had only one wave and no more than inconspicuous ripples thereafter? The stock answer is that in some cities the fall wave infected and immunized so many people that there wasn't enough fresh material to support recurrent waves, Probably so, but this generality, like all others about Spanish influenza, is subject to too many exceptions to be satisfactory. San Francisco had a severe epidemic in October and then another in January.

The factors at work in the pandemic were so numerous and the ways in which they canceled or gained power from one another are so obscure that very few generalities can be drawn. It is true that the disease tended to become less lethal with the passage of time, though the decline was too slow for a week or two or three to make much difference. Flu clearly reached epidemic levels in Seattle a week before it did in San Francisco, but the northern city had an excess flu and pneumonia death rate less than two-thirds that of the southern. To take advantage of the decline in virulency, a community had to lock the door against the disease for many weeks, even months, as did Australia by means of a strict maritime quarantine.

Severe recurring waves of Spanish influenza were characteristic of the South, Middle, and Far West and not of the East, but there are many exceptions to that rule. The pandemic, like many other biological events, was more a thing of particulars than generalities. The states with the highest excess morality rate—Pennsylvania, Montana, Maryland, and Colorado—had little indeed in common economically or demographically, climatically or geographically. . . .

Cities and the Pandemic

What happened . . . to people and families and communities? How did Americans react to Spanish influenza? What did they do to protect themselves? Did the threat drive them apart or did they close ranks and face the danger together?

The answer isn't easy to give because it consists of thousands of separate stories. Shall we therefore examine the stories of a dozen or so individuals? That would be like judging an elephant by examining a dozen cells. Shall we examine the stories of rural areas and small cities? Their chronicles were poorly kept and usually are no more than anecdotal. We are driven to the great cities, which not only kept better statistics on the state of public health than smaller communities, but also published public health reports and had daily newspapers. From these sources we can piece together a narrative of the pandemic in urban America. One obvious danger of using such a sample should be noted: prospective flu victims were packed much more closely together in the cities than in the countryside: they transmitted the disease to one another much more rapidly, and so it is probable that a larger proportion of a city's population would be ill at one time than of a rural or suburban population of the same numerical size. The story of the pandemic in the cities is apt to be more dramatic than elsewhere.

At no time since the widespread application of public health principles in American cities in the last half of the nineteenth century were those cities more ripe for pandemic than in the early years of the twentieth century. In 1911 Lord James Bryce, British ambassador and most widely respected of all living commentators on the United States, published a revised edition of his classic, *The American Commonwealth* wherein he expressed admiration for much about America, but unequivocally announced "that the government of the cities is the one conspicuous failure of the United States." By 1918 the Progressives had made appreciable progress in some cities in ameliorating the conditions that had persuaded Lord Bryce to make such a judgment, but the judgment was still pertinent.

Moralists blamed the cities' troubles on the corruption of individuals, which was, indeed, plentiful, but the primary cause was the immense tide of people flooding into urban centers, both from rural America and the poverty-stricken lands of southern and eastern Europe. Immigrants were especially vulnerable to Spanish influenza because so many of them were young adults.

In 1918 thousands of young men, so recently come from Europe that they weren't yet citizens, were drafted into the army and had to be naturalized in uniform. At the very peak of the flu epidemic in Camp Devense [in Massachussets], Judge Morton of the U.S. District Court had to come into camp to administer the oath of citizenship to 2,300 soldiers, a fairly common event in World War I. The Boston Health Department had to publish its circulars on how to fight flu in Yiddish and Italian, as well as English, and other cities followed suit. One big Pennsylvania mining company issued its antiflu circular in six languages.

The immigrants from rural America had little knowledge of public health principles, but at least could communicate with police, doctors, and nurses. Many foreign immigrants had knowledge neither of public health principles nor English and had little confidence in Protestant, Anglo-Saxon officials, political or medical. This distrust was in part an echo of the strong dislike which native-born Americans felt for immigrants. The self-styled "real Americans" had not yet accepted even the Irish, who had been present in the United States in large numbers for scores of years. A common enough kind of ad for domestic help appearing in the *Boston Evening Transcript* in 1918 read, "A COOK wanted, thoroughly capable, Protestant."

The whole complex of urban problems was exacerbated by the war, as millions more were abruptly summoned into the already crowded cities to manufacture the means to fight the war. Since many of these newest urban immigrants were black, tensions rose which boiled over into a series of race riots, starting with one of the worst in United States history in East St. Louis [Missouri] in 1917 and reaching a peak in 1919.

A misadventure (not typical but useful for illustration) which exemplifies the harmful effects of language and cultural barriers during the pandemic took place at New York City's Municipal Lodging House. Twenty-five Chinese sailors, ill with flu, were brought directly from their ship to the Lodging House, which had been turned into an emergency hospital. There they found themselves among white-cloaked, white-

masked, white people who spoke no Chinese. The only inter-
preter present could not make the sailors understand and,
afraid of infection himself, fled. The sailors refused to take off
their clothing for fear of robbery and refused to eat for fear of
poison. Seventeen of the 25 died.

The case of Johnny B. is an example of what urban alien-
ation could mean, even when there was no language problem.
When Johnny, a fourteen-year-old pneumonia patient, was
ready for discharge from Boston City Hospital, a social worker
checked at his home to see if his family was prepared to receive him. The social worker found the father and two of the
six children ill with influenza. Two other children had died
the previous week. The youngest to die, a baby, had remained
on the kitchen table for three days before the Board of Health
was notified. There was no money because the father was too
sick to work. If the social worker hadn't checked, we may
wonder if anyone would have done so before the rent came
due—and by that time how many would have been alive?

The Health of Children Becomes a Focus of Public Health Systems

Sara Josephine Baker

The earliest efforts of the nation's public health systems concentrated on improving sanitation and combating infectious diseases. Very little attention was paid to the health needs of children until the early 1900s. New York City was the first municipality in the nation to establish a division of child hygiene in 1908. Under the pioneering leadership of Sara Josephine Baker, the bureau established, among other things, a program for the licensing of midwives and the inspection of schoolchildren for infectious diseases. The need for such services in the city was great. New York City had a huge population of poor immigrants who lived in overcrowded and unsanitary conditions.

Sara Josephine Baker studied medicine and graduated from Women's Medical College of the New York Infirmary in New York City. In 1907 she became assistant to the commissioner of health and helped track down Mary Mallon, the notorious carrier of typhoid fever. Baker also developed an approach for preventive health care for children. Her work saw the reduction of infant mortality from 144 per 1,000 live births in 1908 to 66 in 1923. In that year, she wrote a child care manual called The Growing Child. *In it, Baker gave instructions on the hygienic feeding, clothing, and supervision of the young child. Written for the poor, working mother who had little or no education,* The Growing Child *aimed to improve the public health by preventing diseases among the young generation.*

Personal hygiene includes the proper care of the body and its organs so that they may function and develop in a normal manner. Proper personal hygiene is dependent to a great

Sara Josephine Baker, *The Growing Child*. Boston: Little, Brown, 1923.

extent upon the right kind of surroundings, and the normal development of the young child will result not only from the care that is given to the body, but also from the opportunity the child has of living in a clean, decent and wholesome environment.

Cities Are Harmful to Children

The location and general character of the house where the child lives depends upon so many factors that often it is difficult to provide the growing child with exactly the right housing environment. Whenever there is a choice, however, between a crowded city and the more open country, or between a roomy house and a limited apartment, the country and the house should always be chosen.

There are many advantages in city life for children, and statistics have proven only too frequently that country children are not better developed nor more free from disease or physical defects than city children. This is because, as a rule, city children have received more attention not only from their parents but from the community in order to offset the evils of city life, whereas in the country it has been thought that the fresh air and opportunities for outdoor recreation compensated for many defects in feeding, regular hours and proper attention to the care of the skin and the right kind of clothing. These statements are generalities, of course, because individual cases can be cited with the object of proving that country life is the normal one for children. Certainly, no one can seriously question this statement. The physical restrictions of city life are not only burdensome for parents, but they are distinctly harmful for children. Nevertheless, so much depends upon the child's immediate surroundings and environment that there is no reason why children in cities should not have perfect health. This may require attention and care, and a great deal of effort may be necessary to give to the city child the things that come quite naturally to the country child, but, all things considered, the country child has the greatest natural advantages.

Growing children should always have the opportunity for plenty of play space. As a general thing, this is possible only when the family occupies a detached house with a yard or even a greater amount of ground. In addition, the house affords greater opportunities for proper ventilation and plenty of sunshine in the living rooms. The noise, dirt and odors of the city streets are absent. Pure, clean milk and green vegetables are, or should be, fresher and more easily obtainable. With the same amount of care and attention given to the child's life, there is little doubt that the country can be shown to have enormous advantages from the point of view of health.

The Importance of Fresh Air

Growing children need fresh air in abundance. It is absolutely essential for their health. By fresh air is meant not an outing of an hour or so each day, but outdoor life as completely as possible for the entire twenty-four hours. Certainly, the child of preschool age should be able to have most of its recreation in the fresh air except in extremely cold or very stormy weather. In all country climates and where it is possible to have a sleeping porch, the child should be trained to sleep outdoors from the time it is a few weeks old. A porch, preferably one that is above the ground floor, can easily be changed to a sleeping porch. It should be built up on two sides and open on the other two. A roof or awning over the top is advised. The child can be undressed indoors, and, in cold weather, may wear a warm wrapper while going out to bed on the sleeping porch. Sleeping bags made of a steamer rug or heavy woolen blanket will be found useful. These are made by folding the blanket once over and sewing it across one end and partly up one side, leaving an opening at the upper part of the side and across the top. Snap fasteners should be sewed on this opening, and, after the child has been placed in the bag, the latter can be brought together over the shoulders and down the side. Small openings may be made, if desired, so that the hands may be put through. In very cold weather a woolen cap or bonnet is essential, and some warm type of underclothing, such as flannel petticoats or nightdrawers, with knitted socks, should be added. The face is left uncovered but the other parts of the body should be kept warm and the amount of bed covering used should be just sufficient for this purpose.

If, for any reason, the child cannot sleep out-of-doors, the bedroom should be well ventilated. The windows should be open all night. In order to avoid a draft, a window board or window deflector may be used. This may be made at home, and the purpose of its use is to allow free ventilation without drafts. With the window board, the air comes in between the upper and lower sashes; with the window deflector, the air comes directly into the room, but is deflected so that there is no direct air current. A good form of ventilation for the sleeping room, particularly in climates where there are high winds, is to take out one of the upper panes of glass and cover the opening with unbleached muslin. This will give excellent ventilation without draft or marked lowering of the indoor temperature. There should be plenty of bed clothing, and with young children it is permissible to use hot water bottles if there is a tendency for the feet to be cold. The bed should be placed so that there is no direct current of air blowing across it. If necessary, screens should be used.

The human body is usually quite adaptable to its surroundings and people who habitually live in badly ventilated rooms become so accustomed to the close air that they do not seem to notice it, while people coming into the same room from outdoors will be almost stifled. The bad effect of such vitiated atmosphere is particularly marked in children. Children kept indoors in poorly ventilated rooms are almost always pale, underdeveloped and anemic. Usually they suffer from malnutrition, have a poor appetite and are apt to have indigestion. They are almost always constipated. Marked irritability and lack of concentration, with restless sleep, are all indications that the child is not getting enough air. It is probable that sleeping in badly ventilated rooms promotes the growth of adenoids and enlarged tonsils. Certainly, there are few physical defects or varieties of ill-health in children that cannot be caused by lack of fresh air. . . .

The Malnourished Child

Almost always there is bad posture with prominent abdomen and what is known as a "slouchy" attitude. The muscles are soft and flabby, while the hair usually loses its lustre and is dry and brittle. Other symptoms which have to do with the condition of the child may be observed readily. Frequently there is excessive nervousness, with disturbed sleep. There may be twitching of the muscles. The appetite is apt to be diminished, and the child shows marked preference for particular types of food, refusing all others. Undernourished children rarely show any marked vitality. They act as if they were nervously exhausted, do not want to play and are unwilling to make any effort. There is a marked amount of lassitude and fatigue. Any action requires an amount of initiative they are unable to summon. Such children are constantly subject to disease, particularly of an infectious nature.

In order to have effective treatment, it is necessary to interest the child in its own progress. In school children this can be done by means of competition between the various members of the class, to see which will progress most rapidly in weight and general health. With children of preschool age, competition is not so easy to bring about, but even with very young children the sense of personal pride may be brought out in many instances. Each child should have its height measured at least twice a year and should be weighed each month.

A personal weight chart . . . should be used to make an individual record of each case. Progress is the thing to be desired, therefore, the weight curve must have an upward tendency. Any loss of weight or stationary weight for a period longer than one month shows that the type of care given is not suitable.

All insanitary conditions must be eliminated and careful attention paid to the personal hygiene of the child. Many causes of malnutrition have been cured by having the child sleep outdoors or in a room with the windows wide open. Other cases have responded immediately to a course of treatment which included a midday nap or enforced rest for at least two hours a day. Play may have to be restricted to a great extent, particularly if the child is over-active and emotional, and throws itself with all of its energy into every game. Physical defects found to exist must be corrected. Late hours and attendance at the movies must be avoided. The child should have from ten to twelve hours sleep at night and two hours rest in the daytime. Meals must be regular and consist of plain, wholesome food. Feeding between meals is not essential unless the child is not gaining. Then an additional meal of crackers and milk or cocoa may be given in the middle of the forenoon or afternoon and again at night, but this should not be allowed to take the place of the regular meals, and if it interferes with a proper appetite at mealtimes, it should be discontinued. Occasionally, in undernourished children the full value of the food will be more apparent if five small, regular meals a day are given rather than three hearty ones.

There should be a rest period of a half to one hour after each meal during which time the child should lie down out-of-doors or in a well ventilated room, and remain perfectly quiet. Sweets between meals should be forbidden. There is no harm in the sweets themselves; the difficulty is that they usually take away the child's small appetite and make it impossible for it to eat the nourishing diet it needs. Plain candy may be given after meals, but not at any other time. In the dietary, emphasis should be placed upon a full pint and a half of milk a day, plenty of cereals, fresh vegetables, particularly the leafy types, and fruits. Children of preschool age should never, under any circumstances, be allowed to drink either coffee or tea. This is particularly true in regard to the undernourished child.

There is another class of undernourished children that does not respond to any of these types of care. Usually, detailed study will show that the difficulty is with the emotional life of the child. There are instances where children are undernourished, pale and lacking in proper development and the cause is simply the excessive nervous reaction of the child to a disorganized family life. Parental neglect, family discord and an unhappy environment result inevitably in worry and unhappiness to children. Even without harsh punishments, the child can suffer intensely from a sense of general lack of harmony in its environment. Such children are shy and introspective, and inevitably become undernourished. Removal of such a child to a proper environment will result at once in marked improvement.

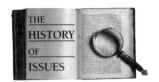

CHAPTER 3

Public Health in the United States, Mid-Twentieth Century to the Present

Chapter Preface

The history of the twentieth century to the opening decade of the twenty-first is notable for increased federal involvement in the nation's public health. In the post–World War II era the health of the environment became a major concern as the federal government legislated on behalf of clean air and clean water. Overt incidents such as the noxious killer-smog that enveloped Donora, Pennsylvania, in 1948 led to the passage of the Clean Air Act. Activists and scientists educated the government and the public on the link between environmental pollution and health and helped bring about landmark legislation such as the Air Pollution Control Act.

Individual initiatives often took the lead in bringing about breakthroughs in combating disease. In the early 1950s, for example, the March of Dimes, the popular name for the National Foundation for Infantile Paralysis, held the largest medical experiment in America's history when it vaccinated 2 million elementary school children against polio. The outbreaks of the disease were halted and the disease was eventually eliminated in the United States. Convincing skeptical parents of the safety of the Salk polio vaccine was the most difficult aspect of the 1954 program. The controversy over vaccination against killer diseases continues, however. In the early twenty-first century the introduction of bills to vaccinate young girls against the virus that causes cervical cancer has stirred arguments among supporters of the vaccination plan and those who oppose it.

The emergence of AIDS in the 1980s as a disease of epidemic proportions among certain groups brought about another series of private and public initiatives. Since then new drugs have evolved to control the spread of AIDS and extend the lifespan of those who are HIV positive. Under current circumstances the nation's public health system must fight a two-front war: one to keep the population from becoming complacent about the danger of AIDS and another to fuel the effort to find a cure.

Prevention of disease continues to be one of the main responsibilities of the nation's public health system. An effort to get the public to avoid or stop smoking has had success among a segment of the population, for example. Yet too many young people, especially young women, continue to take up the habit. Rising body weights among American men, women, and especially children are a current cause for concern. Obese individuals are at risk for comorbid diseases such as heart disease and diabetes, and their medical needs place a huge strain on the health-care system. Federal, state, and local governments are responding to the obesity epidemic in a variety of ways. Municipalities are pressuring restaurants to eliminate the use of transfats in foods and provide more healthful menus. Federal agencies are helping educate Americans about the value of changing their eating habits and increasing physical activity.

The following chapter explores these issues and focuses on how the public health system acts to both teach and pressure Americans to live more healthful lives.

A Deadly Smog Leads to Clean Air Legislation

Lynne Glover

The quality of the air and its impact on the health of the public is a concept that did not enter the consciousness of government until the early 1900s. Noxious fumes from plants and smog were accepted as a fact of life for many living in industrial areas such as Donora, Pennsylvania, a town near Pittsburgh. In October 1948 a temperature inversion settled on the Monongahela Valley towns of Donora and Webster, trapping emissions from local zinc and steel mill smokestacks. As the smog thickened, residents went about their normal routines. On the evening of October 29, the smog became too thick to drive and people walking outside could not see their hands in front of their faces. Air pollution problems at the zinc works were recognized as early as 1918, when the plant owner paid legal claims for pollution that affected the health of nearby residents. The smog in 1948 was different from other incidences of pollution; it was a killer.

Between October 26 and October 31, twenty people were asphyxiated and over seven thousand were hospitalized or became ill as the result of severe air pollution over Donora. The following article was written fifty years after the Donora smog incident and describes what was one of the worst environmental episodes in American history. The investigation of the Donora smog incident gave rise to local, regional, state, and national laws to reduce and control factory smoke and culminated with the passage of the Clean Air Act of 1970. It also marked the beginning of efforts to gauge and deal with the public health threats from air pollution.

Lynne Glover, "Donora's Killer Smog Noted at 50," *Tribune-Review*, October 25, 1998. Reproduced by permission.

In house after house, Bill Schempp placed the mask over the faces of neighbors who were wheezing and gasping for air. He'd give them a little oxygen from the tank, then stop.

They'd start to wheeze again, and the firefighter would give them a bit more. But eventually, it was time to move to the next home in Donora, Washington County [Pennsylvania], to relieve, at least temporarily, the labored breathing of those worst affected by the air pollution that enveloped the town.

"I'm dying, and you're taking my air from me," Schempp, now 81, recalls being told.

Fifty years ago this week, a killer smog created by unchecked industrial emissions and stagnant air conditions filled the then-thriving mill town in the Mon [Monongahela] Valley.

Newspapers reported that 21 people died over two days as a direct result of the smog, and more than a third of the town's population, or about 6,000 people, became ill or were hospitalized.

Victims of the Donora smog will be remembered during a simple memorial service on Wednesday [October 28, 1998]. A representative of the federal Environmental Protection Agency [EPA] will be the guest speaker—significant because of the tragedy's role in shaping today's environmental laws.

"The Donora incident was the dot on the exclamation point on the cry for cleaner air," EPA spokeswoman Ruth Podems said.

No Environmental Controls

Patients with breathing troubles during those last days of October 1948 spilled from examining rooms into corridors at the nearby Monongahela Memorial and Charleroi-Monessen hospitals. The town's community center became an emergency medical station—and temporary morgue.

"This was a great tragedy," said Thomas Ferrall, a spokesman for the U.S. Steel Group of USX Corp. "Environmental control technology that became the norm in our industry didn't exist in 1948."

Emissions from a U.S. Steel Group subsidiary, American Steel & Wire Co., coupled with weather conditions, are the widely accepted causes for the deadly smog. Toxic emissions from the American Steel & Wire's Zinc Works mixed with fog that hung low in the town and lingered because of a common, though unusually long, temperature inversion.

Typically inversions, in which the ground temperature is warmer than the air above, create fogs and last only a few hours. But because there was virtually no wind in the valley, the heavily polluted air remained trapped in the fog for about five days.

"You can't imagine what it was like. You couldn't see your hand in front of your face," said Schempp. The thick, white smoke with its faint odor was like "something out of this world," he said.

During the height of the emergency, the Donora Fire Department was besieged with frantic calls. Soon, help arrived from other communities. The Pitcairn Fire Department arrived with an ambulance, and the McKeesport and Rosedale fire departments loaned inhalators.

Schempp remembers the horrendous time he and a fellow firefighter had attempting to navigate their way on foot through the smoggy Donora streets as they toted 135-pound tanks of oxygen.

For five days, the smog inversion sat over Donora. Newspapers reported that 21 people died over two days.

"It took us at least one hour to go to someone's home only five blocks away," he said. "We had to feel our way along the fence."

With a limited supply, the firefighters could only spare each victim a small amount of oxygen.

Donora is legendary in the annals of environmental history. The incident drew national attention through radio broadcasts at the time, and is discussed today in elementary school science classes and featured in college textbooks.

Sparking the Environmental Movement

For all of its infamy, the tragedy that has been described as the "Hiroshima of air pollution" [referring to the Japanese city on which the first atomic bomb was dropped in World War II] provided the first real piece of scientific evidence in this country that pollution kills.

"It was the first time that anyone looked closely at air pollution and its health effects," said Podems. "It was the first time there was any organized effort to document what happens when air pollutants go above a certain level."

"The Donora smog played a significant role in sparking the environmental movement," said Ken Wolensky, a historian with the Pennsylvania Historical and Museum Commission in Harrisburg. It marked the beginning of government stepping in to examine just what industrial pollution might be doing to people.

At the time, Donora residents didn't know what was happening. "It was something out of this world," Schempp said.

And so life in Donora went on.

The Friday night Halloween parade through town went on as planned. Saturday afternoon's high school football game was played. And the four-mile long mill, which employed 6,500 workers at its peak, continued making zinc, spewing out sulfurous fumes, carbon monoxide, carbon dioxide and heavy metal dusts.

The football game played that weekend may have been one of the greatest games never seen. Although the field was near the top of the hill, where the smog wasn't quite as dense, spectators still could barely see the field. But they could hear the referees' whistles blow.

And they could also hear the announcer call for the children of Bernardo DiSanzi to return home immediately. "I found out later that their dad died," recalled Mayor John Lignelli, 77, who attended the game.

Houseplants and family pets died. And thousands of people suffered severe abdominal cramps, splitting headaches, nausea and vomiting. Strong men and women with no previous health problems were struck down, doctors said, their respiratory systems paralyzed. Elderly people who already had respiratory ailments found themselves choking and coughing up blood.

Autopsy reports of many of those who died indicated "acute changes in the lungs." The victims' ages ranged from 52 to 85.

The town burgess ultimately declared a state of emergency in the town of nearly 14,000. Doctors advised those with respiratory problems to leave town. By Saturday night, however, the heavily congested roads and poor visibility made evacuation impossible.

Those unable to leave were ordered to stay indoors and to make sure their windows and doors remained closed.

And it wasn't until 6 a.m. Sunday that the zinc works was shut down as a precautionary measure.

"The tragic thing was that the residents didn't know what was happening," said Chuck Carson, vice president of environmental affairs for U.S. Steel. "It was only after the fact that they realized 20 people died. Only then did they say, 'Boy, we really had a problem.'"

Pollution was a way of life back then.

Schempp recalled steamboats in the river would regularly blow their horns in order to alert other river traffic of their presence. He said it wasn't unusual for boats to collide because there was so much smoke they couldn't see each other.

"We lived in it. We accepted it," Schempp said of the pollution. He worked in the mill for more than three years and recalls having black ankles when he came home from work. "It was our normal way of life."

But that would change.

"It was on account of what happened here that opened the eyes of the federal government that they needed to do something. Donora should take credit for that," said Lignelli.

No More Donoras

Donora, in fact, can take only part of the credit for an air pollution research bill that was passed in 1955. This was the first federal legislation that mandated the U.S. Public Health Service to conduct research on air pollution effects. It was passed after a 1952 pollution incident in London where more than 1,000 people died.

Donora also helped set the stage for the most ambitious federal environmental law, the Clean Air Act of 1970, which required states to meet and enforce new federal clean-air standards that limited emissions of sulfur dioxide, carbon monoxide, particulate matter and other toxins.

Because of the strict government regulations now in place, Lignelli said he would welcome industry back to Donora, particularly the new Sun Coke Co. [fuel] plant that many residents in the Hazelwood section of Pittsburgh are currently fighting.

"With all the regulations they have now, you probably would not get any smog. For as strict as they are with the Clean Air Act and with all the modern technology that we have today, the air would not bother you at all," said Lignelli.

He added that the Hazelwood residents who point to Donora as a reason to not build the coke plant "are so off base it is pathetic."

For the record, American Steel & Wire Co. formally denied responsibility for the Donora smog, saying it was an "act of God." Still, the company settled hundreds of claims filed by residents of Donora and its downwind neighbor, Webster.

According to U.S. Steel's Ferrall, the out-of-court settlements ranged from $1,000 to $30,000. The 1948 dollar is worth about $7 today, he noted. Many people believe that such an environmental disaster could not happen today.

Harry Klodowski, an environmental attorney who runs a Pittsburgh law firm, said it would be "pretty damn unlikely" that another Donora-like event could occur.

"Factories are not like that anymore," he said. "Nobody has the permission to discharge the kinds of things they were discharging in the 1940s. The regulatory system in place does seem to be working to prevent that kind of thing."

During the Donora smog, emissions of sulfur dioxide were estimated to be somewhere around 1,500 to 5,500 micrograms per cubic meter, said Carson. This is much higher, he noted, than the 80 micrograms per cubic meter average currently mandated by the Clean Air Act.

"We know a lot more now," said Carson. "We have a much sounder scientific basis and much better control systems."

The shutdown of the Donora Zinc Works in 1957, followed by the closure of the entire Steel & Wire Co. operation a decade later, was a devastating blow to the Donora economy.

The population today has dwindled to about 5,000, including some lifelong residents who know nothing about the Donora Smog of 1948. "Never heard of it," said one man strolling through the town.

Polio Vaccine Trials of 1954 Combat a Terrifying Disease

David M. Oshinsky

Polio (short for poliomyelitis) is caused by a virus that enters the body through the mouth, breeds in the intestines, and then circulates in a population through contact with feces. Polio has existed since ancient times but was only totally identified in the early twentieth century by Austrian researchers who determined that it was spread by a virus. This conclusion meant a vaccine against the disease was theoretically possible.

Polio was one of the most feared diseases in industrialized countries because it usually affected children. In 1931 as epidemics broke out in Europe and North America, British researchers identified the three strains of poliovirus, setting off a race to develop a vaccine. The United States led the drive to find a vaccine, thanks in part to the commitment of President Franklin D. Roosevelt, who was paralyzed in both legs by polio at the age of thirty-nine. With Roosevelt's backing, a fund-raising campaign across the United States—the March of Dimes—helped finance the effort.

In 1954, Dr. Jonas Salk of the University of Pittsburgh introduced the first vaccine derived from a "killed" virus. The success of mass trials that year caused an international sensation. Through immunization using this vaccine, the epidemics in North America quickly came to a halt. In the following selection, author David M. Oshinsky describes the Salk vaccine trials of 1954. The trials were unique in the annals of public health because the March of Dimes, the common name of the National Foundation for Infantile Paralysis, independently funded them. As Oshinsky points out, this was in contrast to other diseases such as cancer and heart disease that were receiving government funds to carry on research and conduct trials. The most daunting task of the March of Dimes was convincing skeptical parents to have their children vaccinated.

The Salk vaccine trials of 1954 hold a special, almost reverential, place in the annals of American medicine. Even the most recent articles, written three, four, and five decades after the event, carry titles such as "Making History," "The Shot Heard Around the World," and "The Biggest Public Health Experiment Ever." "The modern era of vaccine evaluation began with the landmark field trial of inactivated poliomyelitis vaccine," said one. "The polio vaccine field trials . . . are among the largest and most publicized clinical trials ever undertaken," said another.

The view from 1954 reflected the same sense of historical excitement. National attention was riveted on the vaccine trials, with news coverage rivaling the other big stories from that remarkable spring. . . . [Jonas] Salk's likeness adorned the cover of *Time* magazine. A Gallup poll showed that more Americans were aware of the field trials than knew "the full name of the President of the United States." By one estimate, two-thirds of the nation had already donated money to the March of Dimes by 1954, and seven million people had volunteered their time. Never before, it appeared, had Americans taken such a personal interest in a medical or scientific pursuit. . . .

Nothing like this had ever been tried before. There were no precedents to follow, no corporate donations to be tapped, no federal assistance. This was virgin territory, the biggest medical gamble in history. The National Foundation for Infantile Paralysis was completely—some thought distressingly—on its own.

That, of course, was the way [March of Dimes chief] Basil O'Connor had envisioned it. Seeing polio as the exclusive territory of the foundation, he had fiercely opposed the "outside interference" of other groups, especially the government, which, he warned, would ensnare the polio crusade in a web of red tape and "socialist thinking." Unlike the American Cancer Society and American Heart Association, which strongly endorsed federal funding for cancer and heart research, the foundation had always lobbied *against* such funding for polio research, describing it, in words reminiscent of Senator Joseph R. McCarthy [who conducted hearings to eradicate Communists], as part of a "Communistic, un-American . . . scheme." So relentless was its message, so powerful was its voice, that others did step aside, leaving the foundation free to pursue its crusade as it, alone, saw fit. At a time when government support for science and medicine was becoming the norm, a top official at the National Institutes of Health told Congress: "We have felt for many years that [the foundation] supports research on such a scale that it would not be wise for us to direct our resources away from other important fields which are not so well covered to this one which is." In that year—1953—the foundation spent about $2 million on polio research; the National Institutes of Health less than $75,000.

Launching the Trials

O'Connor never doubted the foundation's ability to run a major vaccine trial or the public's willingness to support it. Volunteers could easily be mobilized, he thought, and the money could be raised. Indeed, despite a record-breaking $55 million March of Dimes campaign in January 1954, the foundation would conduct its first ever warm-weather appeal in August, raising an additional $20 million to meet the ballooning cost of the trials. There would be some bad blood over this, with a number of cities denying the March of Dimes a solicitor's permit on grounds that it was siphoning too much money away from other worthy causes. O'Connor, naturally, was unmoved. . . .

The vaccine trials would test the National Foundation as never before. Because millions of parents would be asked to risk their children in a potentially dangerous experiment they knew very little about, educating them and easing their fears would be essential. County health officials and school administrators would have to be involved; so, too, medical societies, newspapers, and PTAs. Tens of thousands of volunteers would have to be trained. . . .

Each of the 211 participating counties held a two-day workshop to plan for the trials. Doctors and nurses were briefed about running a vaccine clinic; school principals and teachers about record keeping and contact with parents; chapter volunteers about public participation, including ways to interest "the Negro population." The most delicate issue by far concerned how aggressively children were to be recruited for the trials. Or as the March of Dimes "Discussion Guide" aptly put it, "What pressure should be exerted on parents to get them to sign the request form?"

There was no formal answer. Local counties were expected to meet their quotas with ease. On the one hand, recruiting children was not expected to pose a serious problem in 1954, given the widespread apprehension surrounding the disease. On the other hand, parents needed to know that the trials posed little or no threat, that the risks paled in comparison to the rewards. In the end, it came down to a contest between fear and faith. Americans had long supported the foundation in its effort to end the scourge of polio. Did they trust it enough to put their children on the line?

In a form letter to parents, O'Connor described participation in the trials as a moral act, benefiting not just the volunteers but generations to follow. "This is one of the most important projects in medical history," he wrote. . . .

On the parental consent form, the standard phrase "I give my permission" was changed to "I hereby request," implying that not every child would be fortunate enough to be picked.

The potential risks were aired but quickly dismissed. The ominous-sounding "human experiment" was dropped in favor of "vaccine field study," which had the ring of a benign academic exercise. Parents were told that a killed-virus solution "cannot cause the disease," that the vaccine had been "used safely on over 5,000 volunteers, including Dr. Salk, his wife, and three young sons," that the placebo was a "harmless, but ineffective solution," and that the injections were "only slightly painful" with "no unpleasant effects." So confident was the foundation that it claimed the sole purpose of the trials was "to determine whether the vaccine, *already proved safe*, will give adequate protection against paralytic polio."

Preparing the Vaccine

Before leaving the National Foundation in the fall of 1953, Harry Weaver had made a private deal. Plans for the vaccine field trial were just getting underway. In Toronto, Connaught Laboratories was cultivating large amounts of live poliovirus in a special solution known as Medium 199; in Pittsburgh, Jonas Salk and his staff were busy improving their vaccine. The problem was that Salk had neither the time nor the facilities to turn out the sheer volume needed for the sort of field trial the foundation had in mind. This level of vaccine production would require a commercial source.

In the spring of 1953, Weaver had asked Parke-Davis of Detroit, a major pharmacological house, about its interest in manufacturing Salk's polio vaccine. . . .

For several months, Parke-Davis had the polio vaccine market to itself. Each week, Connaught Laboratories would send a station wagon filled with bottles of live poliovirus across the Canadian border. . . . The process was complex and problems soon arose. Given the urgency, Parke-Davis felt great pressure to move things along. This led to production mistakes that the company blamed on Salk's fault, instructions, and that Salk, in turn, blamed on company error. To make matters worse, Salk was still refining his product, which meant that the advice he provided Parke-Davis was in a constant state of flux. . . .

It was a recipe for trouble. Lacking proper oversight, Parke-Davis found itself unable to reliably duplicate Salk's results. Live poliovirus was discovered in a number of its early batches, leading the foundation to quickly change course. In the fall of 1953 O'Connor invited other pharmaceutical houses to join the vaccine production effort, including Eli Lilly, Wyeth, Sharpe and Dohme, Cutter Laboratories, and Pitman-Moore. . . .

What O'Connor offered these companies was hardly risk free. They would have to build expensive production facilities; the field trials could easily fail; and the vaccine they manufactured would have to be sold at a profit during the length of the trials. Of course, if everything worked out—if the field trials proved successful and the government agreed to license the Salk vaccine for commercial production—these companies would enjoy a financial windfall in the future. The choice was theirs.

Tougher quality controls were also introduced. Each batch of polio vaccine would be triple tested—by the drug firm, by Salk's laboratory, and by the Public Health Service—to assure its safety and potency. . . .

In the end, all of the polio vaccine used in the 1954 field trials was supplied by two pharmaceutical houses—Eli Lilly and Parke-Davis. The latter solved its production problems with the aid of more detailed specifications and more careful quality control. The four other companies—Wyeth, Sharpe and Dohme, Cutter, and Pitman-Moore—would enter the market in the following year, when the government gave the go-ahead for commercial licensing of the Salk vaccine. . . .

The Polio "Shot"

On April 26, at the Franklin Sherman elementary school in McLean, Virginia, six-year-old Randy Kerr stood first in line, sporting a crew cut and a smile. A nurse rolled up his left sleeve; Dr. Richard Mulvaney gave him the injection. "I could barely feel it," boasted America's first polio pioneer. "It hurt less than a penicillin shot."

This procedure was repeated thousands of times in the coming weeks. Each participating school had been assigned a five-member vaccination team that included a doctor who gave the injection, a nurse, a clinic reporter, and two clinic aides. The children were taken to a holding area, where several volunteers (usually classroom mothers) were on hand to keep order. From there, the teacher walked each child to the vaccination room for identification. A clinic reporter entered the date of the shot, looked to see that a parental request form was on file, and checked the lot number of the vaccine. A clinic aide then prepared the child ("rolls up sleeve of left arm to expose triceps muscle; swabs site with an antiseptic on sterile cotton balls"), while the nurse opened the vials of cherry-colored liquid, filled the syringes ("5 cc. syringes will provide five inoculations"), and inserted a new needle after each shot. Before injecting the child, the doctor repeated the lot number to the recorder. A second aide was responsible for disposing of the used syringes, needles, and gauze patches. On the way out, a volunteer handed the child a lollipop. . . .

The field trials were over by late spring, just as the school year ended and the polio season began. And for all the problems encountered, the achievement was immense. More than 600,000 children were vaccinated at least once—two-thirds of whom were in the injected control design and one-third in the observed control design. The most striking statistic was that 95 percent of them had received all three vaccinations, a sign of the intense national publicity, the dedication of local communities, and the devotion of individual parents.

Obesity Among Americans Prompts the Government to Take Action

Rogan Kersh and James Morone

Obesity is an epidemic that threatens the health of Americans and burdens the nation's health-care system. But are obesity and the behaviors that surround it purely a matter of personal choice? Does government have any right to legislate what the public can or cannot eat? Political scientists Rogan Kersh and James Morone address these questions in the following selection.

The authors argue that government has intervened in citizens' private matters on numerous occasions. They examine the historical precedents for government action in personal behavior and identify several conditions that characterize obesity intervention. One of these is social disapproval of the obese; another is demonizing the suppliers of unhealthy foods. As noted by Kersh and Morone the federal government is well on its way to legislating unhealthful foods out of our culture. Efforts to educate children about healthful eating habits have already begun. Public health advocates applaud these efforts but libertarians and the food industry argue that they are nothing more than another example of government meddling in private matters.

Surgeon General David Satcher's 2001 "Call to Action" on obesity begins dramatically: "Overweight and obesity have reached . . . epidemic proportions." Academics, federal officials, medical experts, journalists, and public interest groups have begun to echo the alarm. Unlike most public health problems, however, obesity arises in large part from private behavior: from people's consumption of food and drink. In

Rogan Kersh and James Morone, "The Politics of Obesity: Seven Steps to Government Action," *Health Affairs*, vol. 21, November/December 2002, pp. 142–153. Republished with permission of *Health Affairs: The Policy Journal of the Health Sphere.*

the United States, with its strong culture of individualism, such private activity is often viewed as off-limits to governmental intervention. "The government should stay out of personal choices I make," writes Washington University professor Russell Roberts. "My eating habits or yours don't justify the government's involvement in the kitchen."

Public officials have not yet responded forcefully to the growing concern about an obesity "epidemic." However, the issue—which first met with scornful gibes about "Big Chocolate [a pejorative term for the profitable candy industry]"—has moved onto the U.S. political agenda with remarkable speed. Congress, the White House, and bureaucrats have begun to respond. Will the government eventually regulate fat in the food we eat? In this paper we suggest that it might very well do so. For despite the enduring myths about American self-reliance, the U.S. government has a long tradition of intervening in what seems to be purely private behavior. From alcohol restrictions in the early Republic to the tobacco wars of recent years, personal behavior has regularly become subject to governmental intervention, regulation, and prohibition.

Steps Leading to Political Action

We begin with the historical record. A distinctive set of political conditions generally precedes governmental intervention in the private sphere. We identify seven steps traditionally leading to political action and evaluate which of those steps public health activists have already taken in the obesity case. We then turn directly to government food policy: What is the government actually doing today? What kind of actions might it undertake in the future?

What inspires U.S. public officials to regulate personal behavior? In this section we describe seven "triggers" to action. We developed the triggers by doing our own historical analysis of individual reform movements and then identifying what they shared in common: The following . . . conditions repeatedly characterized public intervention in the private sphere. These triggers do not always operate in a precise cycle; the order and the intensity of each vary with the case. But the politics of public action in at least four ostensibly private areas— drink, drugs, tobacco, and sexuality/family planning— generally includes all the factors.

Social disapproval. The agitation generally begins in society. Observers back to Alexis de Tocqueville [nineteenth-century French political thinker who explored social conditions in America] have commented on the formidable power of social norms and public opinion in the United States. Long before the government stirs, private groups condemn a popular activity. In response to heavy drinking among workers, early-nineteenth-century mill owners and urban elites began to worry about the disruptive effects of alcoholism and preached temperance. In the late nineteenth century men believed that sexual continence was dangerous to their health; large red-light districts flourished in every major city. Victorian feminists rebelled, organized a purity campaign, and set out to close the brothels and change expectations about male behavior.

In these cases, as well as those of illegal drug and tobacco use, the first step to action involves social groups' attacking widely accepted practices. Sometimes the condemnation wins broad support. At other times the criticism is bitterly contested across class, race, gender, or geographic lines. But challenges to private behavior first arise with shifting societal norms.

Obesity has been the subject of powerful public disapproval for more than a century. The criticism developed, quite suddenly, at the end of the nineteenth century. What had long been a mark of prosperity became, as one popular magazine put it in 1914, "an indiscretion, and almost a crime." That view of fat grew stronger over the years (diminishing only during the Depression and world wars). The rise of the diet industry—for which total spending is now estimated at more than $36 billion annually—is one testament to Americans' concern with their weight. A steady stream of reports chronicle widespread antipathy toward overweight people, affecting everything from personal esteem to college admissions and hiring decisions. The first trigger for political regulation of private behavior—social disapproval—has long been tripped in the case of obesity.

Medical science. Public health crusades are typically built on a scientific base. Medical knowledge can rapidly transform society by challenging long-accepted social activities. Early-eighteenth-century Americans, for example, preferred rum and fermented cider to water, which was widely (and often rightly) thought to be unhealthy. As physicians began to issue warnings about alcohol use in the 1830s, Americans' consumption of rum plummeted, falling 75 percent in three decades. In our own time, medical findings about the dangers of tobacco led to concerted pressure against use—and radically transformed consumption habits in little more than a generation.

Although social disapproval of obesity set in during the 1890s, sustained medical concern did not develop for another half-century. This second trigger for government action did not get tripped till the 1950s. Once a medical consensus emerged, the findings spread rapidly. Even so, it took more than two decades for government actors to respond to the health warnings. Public officials did not begin to devote federal resources to publicizing obesity's danger until the 1970s, a development we describe below.

Self-help. In the wake of social sanctions and medical warnings, self-help movements frequently spring up to encourage people to live more healthy lives. This urge, too, is deeply rooted in American history. Urban workingmen in the 1830s founded Washington Temperance Societies to help one another swear off liquor; women formed Martha Washington

Societies, the first female temperance groups. The heirs to these early self-help movements are ubiquitous in modern America. Alcoholics Anonymous is the best-known of thousands of groups, with online "virtual self-help communities" as the latest innovation in this old Yankee tradition.

Obesity organizations stand out in the present-day panoply of self-help. Most such groups target personal behavior—specifically, diet and consumption habits. Some, like Overeaters Anonymous, take on a quasi-religious spirit; others, like Weight Watchers, offer a kind of communal diet program. In short, the third trigger for public action has been activated in the realm of food and obesity since the 1960s, when the first wave of self-help groups for overweight people appeared.

Social disapproval, medical research, and self-help movements are all rooted in the private sector. But together they raise the political salience of health issues. Reformers frustrated by offenders' resistance to their message of uplift and self-improvement urge government sanctions. In the anti-alcohol example, middle-class temperance activists insisted that if people would only take the dry pledge, the mounting troubles facing American cities would become more manageable. In the most enthusiastic dry sermons, urban problems would evaporate entirely. But even with salvation at hand, the incorrigibles refused to take the pledge. They harmed themselves and endangered society. This view of the poor as recalcitrant is no less evident in the present day. And it animates the most troubling trigger (and one of the most powerful) to government regulation of personal behavior.

The demon user. Reformers in all of our cases—drink, drugs, tobacco, and sexual transgressions—urged users to take the pledge, to improve themselves. These misbegotten souls were often people on the social and economic margins: foreigners, racial minorities, the urban masses, and the lower classes. That gave the sermons a racial or class-based edge. Periodically, reformers' disapproval burst into intense social prejudice or demonization.

Who Are the Obese?

Demonizing users—especially poor people minority groups who drink, take drugs, or harbor sexually transmitted diseases—has been one of the most powerful spurs to government action in U.S. history. There is nothing quite like the fear of sinister others to overcome the stalemate of American policy making.

Although overweight Americans have faced popular prejudice for more than a century, critiques of gluttony have not translated into demonization. Antiobesity activists do not portray overweight people as dangerous to society—like drug addicts or smokers polluting the air with secondhand toxins. In part this may be because more than half of U.S. adults are overweight, and nearly one in five is obese. Still, each of the other cases challenged a commonplace activity or condition. In 1965, for example, an estimated 43 percent of American adults were habitual smokers—a figure that has plummeted with changes in social mores, regulatory efforts, and disapproval bordering on the demonization of smokers.

One common thread in past demonization episodes is at least latent in the obesity case. Poor people and members of minority groups tend to be more obese than other Americans are. Given the historical patterns of other ostensibly private consumption practices, the opportunity for demonization may well be present. But, to date, this has not been taken up by those calling for action against obesity.

Demon industry. In all four of our comparative cases, activists attack the producers or suppliers. They charge corporate villains with seeking profits by peddling poison. Worse, the greedy industry lures children into destructive habits. The contemporary tobacco case is typical—a ruthless industry unleashes Joe Camel to ensnare America's youth. . . . Similarly, the drug peddler lurking near the schoolyard offers a classic twentieth-century icon of malice. Together, demon users and malevolent industries have been powerful triggers to political action across U.S. history.

For unhealthy foods and obesity, this trigger emerged into political play in, roughly, 1999. The fast-food industry has become the most visible target. Eric Schlosser's surprise bestseller, *Fast Food Nation*, featured some familiar demonization arguments: A cynical industry targets children, reshapes their eating habits (it is hugely "profitable to increase the size and the fat content of their portions"), and literally sponsors an epidemic ("no other nation in history has gotten so fat so fast"). Schlosser further blames the industry for a long list of harms: It has trashed the American countryside, widened the gap between rich and poor, reconstructed the entire meatpacking industry (his details of working conditions are as horrifying as anything in Upton Sinclair's *The Jungle*), and cynically fed an obesity epidemic. The result is "emotional pain," "low self-esteem," and widespread illness and death. Until Schlosser's book achieved best-selling status, critics of any segment of the food industry had not found a wide audience, either in the general public or among policymakers. But a growing literature slams fast foods, junk foods, and soft drinks....

From a Private Health Matter to a Political Issue

With this trigger in cultural play, obesity begins to shift from being a private health matter to being a political issue. Scientific findings never carry the same political weight as does a villain threatening American youth. If critics successfully cast portions of the industry in this way, far-reaching political interventions are possible, even likely. When an industry becomes demonized, plausible counterarguments (privacy, civil liberties, property rights, and the observation that "everyone does it") begin to totter.

In any case, obesity politics now centers on this trigger. Critics have begun the attack (and have launched what is likely to be a substantial flock of related lawsuits). Two additional triggers will help to determine how far the critics get.

Organizing to Fight Obesity

Identify a looming evil, and Americans often organize movements demanding a response. Activists, grouped en masse, can cut through barriers to political action by seizing the attention of policymakers. When small numbers of women knelt in prayer outside saloons in the 1870s, they met with derision. When the Women's Christian Temperance Union (WCTU) got 200,000 women fighting liquor—the first women's mass movement in the United States—they were welcomed into meetings with political leaders. Mass movements trigger political action. . . .

Obesity politics has never stirred popular awareness on the order of WCTU marches against alcohol or the "Just Say No" antidrug crusades. When the *New Republic* published a supportive profile of a prominent advocate of government-sponsored antiobesity regulation, Yale psychologist Kelly Brownell, it emphasized the lack of popular agitation: "Brownell is not out leading a mass movement on the streets of New Haven and has no plans to do so." However, demonization generally precedes mobilization: The politics of the preceding trigger will affect the prospects for this one. If supersizing a soft drink and fries begins to seem as dangerous as lighting up a cigarette, a movement may very well spring up. . . .

Interest-group action. Cultural images ("Big Tobacco," "Just Say No") and mass movements win political attention. Interest groups translate popular energy into specific complaints and detailed policy proposals. In the antialcohol struggle, the WCTU got the attention. . . .

On the obesity front, public health groups such as the American Heart Association (AHA) and the National Cancer Institute (NCI) have advocated efforts to improve dietary habits since 1952, when the AHA identified obesity as a major cardiac risk factor and promoted low-fat, low-cholesterol diets and increased exercise as a response. More recently, critics of the food industry, such as the Center for Science in the Public Interest (CSPI), have mounted anti-obesity campaigns in and beyond Washington. One of the nation's largest health care philanthropies, the Robert Wood Johnson Foundation, recently joined the fray in defining lifestyle (including tobacco use and obesity) as one of its major concerns. . . .

Although social scientists often depict the U.S. government as relatively weak, it has been far more ready than most Western regimes have been to regulate (or prohibit) private behavior. The politics of social control generally feature the . . . triggers discussed here. Of course, political history does not permit causal claims, but we believe that these descriptive analogies across time and issue areas offer a useful policy guide. . . .

Feeble Responses to Food Consumption

Political efforts to curb obesity will likely generate considerable debate, and perhaps action, in the future. For the present, however, governmental food policies tilt in a very different direction. Public regulation of high-fat foods has been limited to ensuring purity and, more recently, promoting nutrition. On the other hand, both local and national governments have actively encouraged the production and consumption of high-fat foods, especially meat and dairy products. The next sections review governmental activity in this realm over the past century.

Purity. Although an antifat culture had begun to stir in the 1890s, the central political issue was food purity. Sinclair's *The Jungle* generated enough public outrage to overcome industry opposition, and after several false starts Congress passed a Pure Food and Drug Act along with a permanent federal appropriation for meat inspection (both in 1906). . . .

Today governmental action remains more focused on purity and accuracy than on nutritional value. In 1999 a consortium of governmental, academic, and commercial weight-loss organizations developed new consumer-information guidelines about commercial diet programs. The Federal Trade Commission (FTC) has also been investigating fraudulent or misleading diet claims. Although critics are not yet satisfied with food inspection standards, federal attention to purity and fair market practices far exceeds attention to obesity and unhealthy foods. And compared with governmental control of alcohol, drugs, and tobacco, the response to food consumption has been feeble.

Advertising fat's dangers. . . . The federal government did not officially acknowledge the connection between diet and the risk of chronic disease until 1969, when at White House conference was held on food, nutrition, and health. Subsequent action has focused primarily on collecting information, disseminating findings, and sponsoring further research. While these are not normally controversial activities, in food politics they have generated much heat. Take the apparently innocuous topic of food labeling. It was authorized by Congress in 1906 (as part of the Pure Food and Drug Act) and strongly recommended in a 1938 statute, the Food, Drug, and Cosmetic Act. The Food and Drug Administration (FDA) launched a voluntary labeling program in 1973. Prodded by the states, especially California and New York, Congress finally mandated labeling in 1990—although implementation delays dragged on until 1994. . . .

Regulation. Federal and state actors have been deeply involved in the production, distribution, and consumption of food. The U.S. Department of Agriculture (USDA) was established during [Abraham] Lincoln's presidency, with nutritional issues today overseen by it and myriad agencies and departments, including the FTC; the U.S. Department of Commerce; and a number of units within the U.S. Department of Health and Human Services (HHS), including the FDA, the National Institutes of Health (NIH), and many others. . . .

Government Support for Fatty Foods

Regulating high-fat, low-nutrition foods—again, partial culprits behind rising obesity rates—seems particularly difficult, given the complexity of the food regime. However, perhaps as a result of increasing attention to obesity and the first signs of industry demonization, a regulatory regime has begun to emerge. Before reviewing that development, we look at government action that appears to sustain, and even encourage, rising American obesity rates.

Aiding and abetting. Instead of controlling high-fat foods, government policy actively supports them—sometimes at the expense of low-fat alternatives. The three primary sources of fat in the typical American diet are red meat, plant oils, and dairy products. Producers of all three are subsidized or otherwise aided by federal, state, and local authorities. At times the state goes further and promotes fatty foods. Surplus high-fat dairy products, for example, have long been a mainstay of federal nutrition assistance programs, including the NSLP [National School Lunch Program]. The USDA pursues what [nutrition scholar Laura] Sims tags a "schizophrenic mission." The agency supports beef producers "while issuing dietary guidance about meat consumption." Official policy choices may only inadvertently encourage fatty American diets, but this contribution is rarely acknowledged. "The 'politics of fat,'" concludes Sims, "has been conspicuously absent from debates over agricultural policy."

Steps Government Might Take

If the federal government were to mobilize against obesity, what might it do? Governmental policies toward alcohol, tobacco, and drugs include at least four regulatory strategies: controlling the conditions of sale through direct restrictions or limits (especially aimed at youth); raising prices through "sin taxes"; government litigation against producers of unhealthy substances with damage awards earmarked for health care or healthy alternatives; and regulating marketing and advertising. As we noted above, federal officials already promote alternatives to unhealthy eating, via education programs warning consumers about health risks; stronger education measures might include government-funded cessation programs addressing compulsive behavior, or direct subsidies for healthy alternatives. A combination of these policies—now in place at state and federal levels for tobacco, alcohol, and drugs—could be applied to unhealthful, low-nutrition foods. . . .

If American history is any guide, rising social disapprobation, conclusive medical knowledge, and further criticism of industry (perhaps alongside attacks on obese individuals) may fan the flame of interest-group activity—including litigation—and result in far more government regulation of fatty foods. Such sanctions would represent a nightmare for libertarians and the food industry. To many public health advocates, they constitute necessary protection against what one writer terms "North Americans' sedentary suicide." For now, the political battle has been joined.

A City Meets the Diabetes Crisis by Monitoring Blood Glucose Levels

Joyce Frieden

Along with obesity, its comorbid condition, diabetes has become an American disease of near epidemic proportions. Nearly 21 million American children and adults have diabetes, but only two-thirds have been diagnosed. Another 54 million have pre-diabetes. While diabetes is a manageable disease, an individual's ability to effectively manage it is directly connected to his or her ability to access and use appropriate health care. Without access to diabetes medications, equipment, and educational training, people with diabetes are at a much greater risk for diabetes-related complications such as blindness, kidney failure, and amputations. Needless to say, the poor are more likely to suffer from complications and succumb to death as a result of uncontrolled or undertreated diabetes.

With one of the largest diabetic populations in the nation, New York City's public health system faces great challenges in dealing with the disease. Noncompliance on the part of the diabetic is one of the main stumbling blocks. As author Joyce Frieden points out in the following article, the city has taken the extreme measure of having laboratories report the results of blood tests to the health department. By doing so, the health department is better able to monitor diabetics and keep them actively involved in their treatment. While the program raises important issues of patient privacy, physicians and public health officials see the benefits of monitoring programs outweighing the disadvantages.

A diabetes monitoring program starting last month [January 2006] in New York City is drawing praise while also raising questions about confidentiality.

Under the program, clinical laboratories now send the results of all hemoglobin tests that they run to the health department.

As the program develops, the health department will provide information to clinicians on their patients with diabetes, as well as contact those patients whose results indicate poor glycemic control. "Poor control" has yet to be defined but will be determined by analysis of initial patient data.

Such contact letters—sent to patients as well as their doctors—could explain what the test results mean and could offer advice on how to achieve better control. Eventually, the health department also may provide more intensive services to those with the highest levels.

The goals are to "understand the epidemic better, and understand the level of glycemic control in the population" and also to see if better monitoring will help improve diabetes outcomes, according to Dr. Lynn Silver, assistant commissioner for chronic disease prevention and control at the city's Department of Health and Mental Hygiene.

In New York and across the nation, it's been demonstrated that certain quality improvement tools, such as registries, can improve diabetes care, she added.

Family physicians should welcome the opportunity for public health officials to help them with diabetes patients, said Dr. Neil Calman, president of the Institute for Urban Family Health, in New York. "My sense is that the people who are out of control for the most part are out of control because they haven't fully engaged in their treatment program. So having the assistance of public health officials to help engage them in treatment is important," he noted in an interview.

"Public health has to be viewed beyond the traditional confines of infectious disease, and just as we would expect the health department to intervene in an epidemic of an infectious disease like influenza or some other epidemic, diabetes has become this type of epidemic in New York City, and in fact is responsible for more morbidity and mortality than many infectious diseases."

"Hopefully, [this] will become a model for the rest of the country," he said.

A Place to Wage War Against Diabetes

New York City is the quintessential place for waging such a public health–led war on diabetes. According to surveys, the prevalence of self-reported diabetes shot up from 3.9% in 1993 to 9% in 2003, or to 530,000 people. And if one factors in those not yet diagnosed, the number of New Yorkers with diabetes is closer to 750,000, according to Dr. Silver.

"Most practices can't tell you who their diabetes patients are and how they're doing unless they have a very well organized electronic health record. There have been a number of studies showing that just to know who diabetes patients are and monitoring how they are doing can be a really helpful step in efforts to improve quality. This will give us an important intervention to provide support to practitioners," she added.

But some physicians don't seem to want the help. "If the test shows an undesirable result, what are doctors going to do about it?" said Dr. Jane Orient, executive director of the Association of American Physicians and Surgeons, Tucson, Ariz. "A lot of this is out of my hands, a patient may say, 'I've got better things to do. I'm not going to test my blood six times a day.' Or 'I know I need to lose weight, but I'm not going to do it.' For a lot of diabetics, it's not possible to control them because it depends so much on patient behavior."

Others think that the program is a good idea. "This should significantly help in the improvement of diabetes control, both for patients and clinicians," Dr. Allan Rosenfield, dean of the Mailman School of Public Health at Columbia University, New York, wrote in a letter to the health department. "I think this is an important step forward."

Dr. Steven Safyer, chief medical officer of Montefiore Medical Center, New York, agreed. "The need is urgent," he said in a letter. "Montefiore wholeheartedly supports putting in the hands of the health department the information it needs to help patients and clinicians better manage this devastating chronic disease."

One issue that is foremost for many people is confidentiality, since the database is not anonymous. "I'm concerned about the government having information about their status as chronic disease patients in an electronic format, which could lead to discrimination if it gets out," Dr. Orient said. And the likelihood of the information getting inadvertently released is high, since it's not secure, she said.

Dr. Silver disagreed: "We've been collecting confidential data on sensitive issues for 100 years without any significant breaches of confidentiality," she said. "While we recognize these can be legitimate concerns, we feel the potential benefit in light of the epidemic condition outweighs any risk to privacy."

Patients will be able to opt out of the intervention phase of the program, but not out of the data collection phase, Dr. Silver said. The opt-out opportunity will come when the patient first receives the letter about the test results; the opt-out will remain available after that.

Although concerns about privacy are important, Dr. Calman said the issue is one that is manageable. "It's not a 'domino theory' where if you give the health department access to the patient's hemoglobin the entire record will become available soon."

Dr. Paul Jellinger, immediate past president of the American College of Endocrinology, said privacy issues are always a concern for diabetes patients.

Protecting a Patient's Privacy

New York officials "need to take great care in making certain that the individual's privacy is protected because once one loses that protection, being branded a poorly controlled or uncontrolled diabetic can have significant ramifications, insurance-wise or employment-wise," said Dr. Jellinger, who is also professor of medicine on the voluntary faculty of the University of Miami and in practice at the Center for Diabetes and Endocrine Care in Hollywood, Fla.

But as long as the privacy issues are properly managed, "the idea of tracking diabetics is a good one," he continued. Dr. Jellinger noted that a 39-state study done by the American Association of Clinical Endocrinologists found that 67% of patients had hemoglobin levels greater than 6.5%, the organization's recommended target for good control of diabetes. "I like the idea that someone is going to monitor patients because it brings home the finding of the study that a lot of people are not aware they aren't reaching the goal," he said.

The thing that will really make the difference, though, is the intervention piece, Dr. Jellinger said.

"Giving patients a gentle nudge or pestering them—that's not the way to do it. The nature of the intervention needs to be effective; it has to be something meaningful. It needs to be more time with a physician, funding for diabetes education, and counseling by a dietician," Dr. Jellinger said. He suggested that the city consider setting up clinics for diabetes patients to get this kind of help.

Dr. Silver said that the city is still designing the interventions, which will start in the second year of the program. (The first year will just involve collecting and analyzing the data.) As a model, the city is looking at the Vermont Diabetes Information System, "which uses a voluntary reporting system combined with automated feedback to physicians," she explained.

"It generates a quarterly report to physicians on all their patients with diabetes and classifies them on how they're doing. It also provides information to patients, which goes out under the physician's name."

Dr. Silver emphasized that the Vermont program "goes out in a way to support care to patients, and not interfere [with the physician-patient relationship]." For instance, patients overdue for a test get a letter from the system on behalf of their doctors. The city is also studying "more robust" disease management to support the people who are doing the worst, she said.

The city hopes to have a pilot intervention program up and running by next year [2007], according to Dr. Silver. The pilot will probably be done in South Bronx, which has a diabetes prevalence of 18% among adults, she said.

Vaccine for Human Papillomavirus Causes Controversy

Rita Rubin

The development of vaccines against infectious diseases is one of the great achievements in the history of public health in the twentieth century. By vaccinating children against diseases such as polio and diphtheria, the public health system added at least twenty-five years to the life expectancy of Americans. At the beginning of the twentieth century, infectious diseases were widely prevalent in the United States and exacted an enormous toll on the population. According to the Centers for Disease Control, in 1920 alone nearly 470,000 measles cases were reported and 7,575 patients died. Today, measles has been nearly eradicated in the United States. Yet other maladies such as human papillomavirus, or HPV, have arisen to take the place of these earlier scourges.

A vaccine has been developed to combat HPV and is approved by the Food and Drug Administration (FDA) for use. The existence of a vaccine is no assurance that it will ever be used, however. There is a debate over whether or not state governments should mandate vaccinating the female population against this sexually transmitted disease and a leading cause of cervical cancer. That debate reveals the ongoing issue of the government's right to protect the public health versus the rights of the individual parent to decide what is right for his or her child and is the topic of the following selection. As in previous eras, there are some Americans who are opposed to vaccination programs on religious grounds or their rights as parents to have authority over their children. They are against mandatory immunization. Some members of the medical community are also divided about the wisdom of mandating a vaccine against HPV. As author Rita Rubin writes, they prefer public education programs to convince wary citizens of the value of the vaccine.

A sk nearly anyone whether vaccinating girls against cervical cancer is a good idea, and you're likely to get an affirmative reply.

Ask whether states should require girls to get vaccinated, though, and you're likely to get more varied answers. But you might be surprised about who falls on which side.

The debate over mandating vaccination against human papillomavirus, or HPV, which causes cervical cancer, has heightened since Republican Texas Gov. Rick Perry issued an executive order Friday [February 2, 2007] requiring girls to be immunized before entering sixth grade, as of September 2008. Parents can opt out for reasons of conscience.

Legislators in 23 states and the District of Columbia have introduced bills to mandate HPV vaccination, according to Women in Government, a national, bipartisan organization of female state legislators that is pushing for mandatory immunization. The group ... attracted criticism because it has received unrestricted educational grants from HPV vaccine maker Merck, which stands to profit greatly from state mandates.

The vaccine, called Gardasil, targets two types of HPV—a sexually transmitted infection—that cause 70% of cervical cancers, and two types that cause 90% of genital warts cases.

Even before the vaccine won Food and Drug Administration approval last June, there were objections to making it mandatory. And Concerned Women for America, which, its website says, strives to "bring Biblical principles into all levels of public policy," issued this response to Perry's order: "Concerned Women for America believes that it is the right and responsibility of parents—not government—to choose whether or not their daughter receives the vaccination."

Parents Can Opt Out

In a statement . . . , Perry said, "I am a strong believer in protecting parental rights, which is why this executive order allows them to opt out."

Columbia University public health researcher James Colgrove says every state except West Virginia and Mississippi allows parents to opt out of getting their children vaccinated on religious grounds. But, Colgrove wrote in December in *The New England Journal of Medicine*, "it is a mistake . . . to view the contrasting stances on HPV-vaccine mandates as solely, or even primarily, evidence of a conflict between science and religion."

In an interview . . . , Colgrove said mandating HPV vaccination could lead to a backlash that would result in fewer girls getting immunized. Perry's order, "if anything, will help to mobilize opposition," he said. "You have to consider it in the context of the already long list of vaccines that children are required to get."

By rushing to mandate HPV immunization, says Samuel Katz, a co-developer of the measles vaccine, "you just throw oil on the flames of the anti-vaccine folks." The measles vaccine, licensed in 1963, launched the debate about mandating immunizations, Katz, pediatrics professor emeritus at Duke University, said Wednesday. But HPV isn't the measles, he says. "It isn't transmitted in a classroom to dozens of children. It's not the same thing as infectious diseases that fly through the air with no boundaries."

There is still much to be learned about the proper use of the HPV vaccine, Katz says. "When you start with a new vaccine, you have to go through a period of public education, as well as health-worker education," Katz says. "I think eventually this (HPV immunization) will spread to the population at large, but I don't think the way to get there is to mandate."

Dartmouth doctor Diane Harper, an investigator in clinical trials of Gardasil and Glaxo's not-yet-approved HPV vaccine, says she worries that mandating immunization will create a false sense of security that may cause women to skip Pap smears. "The vaccine is not a silver bullet, is not a shield against cancer."

Mark Einstein, director of clinical research for gynecological oncology at Montefiore Medical Center in New York, believes it should be mandated, but "we weren't expecting anything to happen so soon." With more education, he says, "people will realize this is just another method" to prevent cervical cancer.

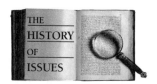

CHAPTER 4

Global Public Health
Challenges for the Future

Chapter Preface

The achievements of America's public health system during the past century are impressive. Improved sanitation and hygiene coupled with the discovery of antibiotics did much to eliminate old diseases such as cholera. The implementation of universal vaccination programs led to the elimination of childhood diseases such as measles, diphtheria, and polio and added at least twenty-five years to the lifespan of Americans. The victory over infectious diseases is still not won, however.

The nation's public health system must address the emergence of new infectious diseases. These include such diseases as severe acute respiratory syndrome, or SARS, the reemergence of old diseases such as tuberculosis, outbreaks of diseases that can be traced to tainted foods, and acts of bioterrorism. Meeting these challenges will require improved systems of disease surveillance and response at the local, state, and federal levels. Because diseases can quickly leap across national borders, global communication and outbreak response must also be improved. Border areas between nations, especially where people are poor, live in environmentally toxic settings, and have little or no access to basic health care, are particularly vulnerable to outbreaks of disease. International communication and cooperation will be essential in a time of pandemic.

In the meantime our public health system continues to carry on research on the possible role of infectious agents in causing or intensifying certain chronic diseases. These include diabetes, some cancers such as the human papillomavirus and heart disease. While scientific work goes on in the laboratory in search of cures, public health departments continue to use a battery of methods to encourage citizens to take active roles in their own health. Information about specific diseases or health issues is now easily accessed via the Internet from federal, state, and local agencies. The public health departments of large cities reach out to groups at risk for diseases such as diabetes by funding free testing or monitoring programs. Schools are taking a proactive role by changing menus to include more healthful foods and developing physical education programs geared to all students.

The following chapter examines some global public health challenges for the coming years. It asks some important questions: Will our public health system be prepared in the event of another terrorist attack? How will the nation's health system deal with the long-term needs of severely wounded and disabled war veterans? How will climate change affect the lives of generations to come? And how do we address some persistent problems such as unequal access to health care?

Learning from September 11, 2001, to Prepare for the Future

David Rosner and Gerald Markowitz

The terrorist attacks of September 11, 2001, or 9/11, made it apparent that public health agencies and those who work in them are vital components of a nation's response to disasters. That conclusion inspired authors David Rosner and Gerald Markowitz to write a book about the experiences of public health workers in New York City who had been involved in the response to 9/11. In the following selection from Are We Ready? *Rosner and Markowitz note the importance of city agencies, laboratories, hospitals, and personnel that, taken together, form the public health infrastructure. They also point to the need for clear lines of authority in times of crisis. In addition, Rosner and Markowitz argue on behalf of expanding the notion of what constitutes dangers to the public health. In the midst of our current war on terrorism, state and local authorities fear that there will not be enough money to pay for both expanded police and fire departments and traditional public health sectors not tied to emergency preparedness or bioterrorism.*

David Rosner is a professor of history and public health at Columbia University and director of the new Center for the History of Public Health at Columbia's Mailman School of Public Health. He is author of A Once Charitable Enterprise *and editor of* Hives of Sickness: Public Health and Epidemics in New York City. *In addition, he has coauthored and edited with Gerald Markowitz, a distinguished professor of history at the City University of New York, numerous books and articles, including* Deadly Dust: Silicosis and the Politics of Occupational Disease in Twentieth-Century America.

Much of the success of the public health response to 9/11 [the September 11, 2001, terrorist attacks] in New York City had less to do with formal emergency planning or conscious preparation than with the presence of an existing infrastructure of health services, laboratories, and personnel. Though many officials outside the city praised New York's ability to take action during the crisis, and some personalized its success by attributing it to the political leadership, in fact the work was done by bureaucracies that nothing and no one could have mobilized had they not already been there.

Lessons Learned from New York City's Response

A second major lesson of New York City's experience is that we need to develop a more expansive understanding of mental health services and integrate our current, individualized system more broadly into our public health infrastructure. In fact, on July 1, 2002, the city's Department of Health merged with the Department of Mental Health to become the Department of Health and Mental Hygiene. It becomes clear, once we acknowledge the broad impact of terrorism on the mental health of society, that all people affected—from schoolchildren in the immediate area of the attack on the World Trade Center to their parents, neighborhood residents, and anyone directly touched by the tragedy—deserve comprehensive mental health care, regardless of their income or private insurance coverage. This recognition has the potential to lead to a huge transformation in how we conceive of our society's responsibilities to those in need. Whether this challenge to our broader assumptions about who is "worthy" and who is "unworthy" of care will gain strength or will fade remains to be seen. An ancillary point is that we need a much better understanding of how best to respond to a population's social and economic needs in a crisis. The public health and social welfare communities initially responded to the trauma of 9/11 by abandoning practices of the past decades—indeed, the past century—that had often inhibited access to a variety of services. Immediately following the attack, a more open system of social services was instituted. However, this early promise of broader rights to health and social welfare services, irrespective of income, was soon lost.

A third message that comes through loud and clear is that failure to communicate honestly about uncertainty is a big mistake. The issuance of pronouncements that obviously are not supported by everyday observations will in the end backfire, as the public officials making such claims are certain to lose the public's trust and goodwill and ultimately their authority. Human beings will persist in believing that air that smells and makes us cough is not good for us, no matter what experts or political leaders say about the lack of danger as indicated by scientific investigations.

Finally, the attacks of September 11, 2001, were on the nation, not just New York City, the Pentagon, or Pennsylvania. When national threats are present, clear lines of federal and other authority need to be established. A cacophony of voices does not serve the public well or use resources efficiently. Local authority need not be usurped, but decisive leaders who control resources and make decisions with good personal and situational intelligence are required in times of crisis. In the anthrax event, where there was clear leadership (e.g., that of Mayor Rudy Giuliani), the system worked reasonably well. When many jurisdictions operated within their narrow preserves, communicating poorly and competing for primacy, the system fell apart.

The Concept of Public Health Must Expand

In examining the public health community's response in the various states, we conclude that even as "emergency response" is in the process of being defined, the purview of public health must continue to expand, helping professionals in the field to understand the breadth of social and medical activities that determine a population's health and well-being. For much of the past century, public health officials, politicians, and administrators of city agencies in general clung to very traditional notions of what constituted dangers to the public's health, which they addressed in discrete functions: sanitation, emergency care, scientific data collection, and surveillance. But in recent decades this narrow definition of public responsibility began to give way, a process accelerated considerably by the events of the past five years, which have forced government officials—indeed, all of us—to rethink what health is, which agencies are responsible for a population's health, and what the public's role is in defining an environment as healthful or unhealthful.

In response, government officials at the state and local levels paid attention to a broad array of social service, public health, and health care needs, each with its claim on scarce state and federal resources. Public health officials focused on the possibility of improving the traditional infrastructure of their agencies, including lab capacity, surveillance systems, lines of intra- and interagency communication, and processes for protecting the borders. Certainly, the mobilization around public health needs led to the allocation of significant resources and to what many of those to whom we spoke called "progress." After September 11, 2001, officials and legislators in state government were buttered by geopolitical events and federal decisions that dramatically altered the basic assumptions under which they had long operated. Rural country officials, often isolated and laboring far from state as well as federal seats of power, could hardly be expected to be fully prepared for their new responsibilities for developing plans to defend against a bioterrorist or chemical attack. At the state level, legislators and officials responsible for population health and well-being had to attend to an extensive array of needs at a time when resources were scarce.

New Resources vs. Balanced Budgets

In the early months after the attacks and the anthrax episodes, those concerned about public health in America believed that the new resources supplied by the federal government could be used to address long-standing infrastructure weaknesses as well as to meet the new antiterrorism mandates. State officials were accustomed to some "cause of the day" receiving massive funding for a year or two and then being forgotten, but they believed that this time it would be different, that the profound shock of 9/11 would lead to equally profound changes. Many state officials anticipated that the federal government would finally fund public and population health programs at a level that would protect citizens not only from narrowly defined bioterrorist threats but also from SARS [severe acute respiratory syndrome] and other infectious diseases. Some even hoped for general improvements in health care and the availability of health insurance. There was no intrinsic contradiction between the traditional goals of public health departments—such as investigating and monitoring illnesses, studying them in the laboratory, and providing well-baby services and health care for the uninsured—and the new goal of participating as full members in an emergency response team. Officials in general government and those in public health agencies agreed on many of the same goals—but state legislators and their staffs had to create balanced budgets that devoted about 80 percent of their expenditures to entitlement programs (such as Medicaid), whereas those in public health agencies sought to maintain programs more traditionally associated with preventive services.

Media coverage, our interviews, and reports both published and unpublished make clear that in the years since 9/11, much has been done to provide more resources, begin needed legal reform, improve surveillance, and enhance communications. The focus of the Centers for Disease Control and Prevention (CDC) and Health Resources and Services Administration programs has expanded beyond smallpox and preparations for war against Iraq, while their grant programs demonstrate that the federal government remains committed to addressing all forms of terrorism: the amounts awarded in fiscal years 2003, 2004, and 2005 match those in 2002. The strengthening of the public health infrastructure (together with employment growth as the country recovers from a recession) has resulted in a modest improvement in access to health care, general childhood inoculation programs, well-baby services, and mental health care. It has also aided the co-ordination of emergency response within and between agencies; in some communities, laboratory capacity has improved. According to the CDC, federal initiatives, grants, and programs have resulted in a number of significant improvements in public health preparedness within individual states.

The Role of the CDC

Through its own grants, the CDC has fostered the development of surveillance systems, management information systems, interagency cooperative agreements, and twenty-four-hour-a-day public health emergency response systems; it has also identified physicians who, in an emergency, will serve as consultants in diagnosing and treating infectious diseases. Among its accomplishments are stronger relationships between law enforcement officers and health providers, enhanced epidemiological and laboratory capacity, better training for possible bioterrorist events, improved and more secure communication systems, and successful inoculation of a group of health professionals who are now capable of responding to a smallpox outbreak. Joseph Henderson, a CDC senior management official, notes, "In 2005, CDC will be awarding $862,777,000 to support state and local public health response efforts. Since these funds are intended to enhance detection and surveillance capabilities, improve laboratory diagnostic capacities, improve the delivery and quality of workforce training, improve outbreak control and containment strategies, and enable improved communication, it goes without saying that the basic public health infrastructure benefits from these investments."

Certain bioterrorism-specific reforms will undoubtedly remain, but the early optimism fueled by new federal interest and funding has waned as state legislators, governors, and public health officials all have come up against state and federal budget crises and a falloff of federal attention. Legislators in most states have had to make hard choices in allocating their reduced monies for education, social welfare, direct health services, and population health more generally. Real funding increases are needed to build up the public health infrastructure sufficiently for these departments to shoulder the new burden of countering terrorism and bioterrorism. Many public health officials were bitterly disappointed that the apparent federal commitment to these upgrades vanished as memories of September 11 began to fade. The nation's public and population health infrastructure unquestionably has suffered as a consequence of the Bush administration's repeated insistence to the nation that Iraq was the focal point of the real war on terrorism—and therefore of our budget priorities. And many perceived a schism between those who favored a narrow focus on smallpox and those who argued for building up defenses against bioterrorism in general and strengthening long-term population health. As Dennis Perrotta [state epidemiologist] of Texas points out, "The small pox vaccination effort in many jurisdictions was seen as a distraction from basic preparedness and public health activities. The growth of this area seemed incongruent with the significant losses of population health programs as states and state health departments faced fiscal conditions of unparalleled instability."

Is Health an Adjunct to National Defense?

State officials vary in their confidence that their states will be able to ride out the budget problems currently hobbling their public and population health programs. Further, some are concerned that in the long run, emergency preparedness will be impaired by a weakened public health system. Michael Caldwell, commissioner of the Dutchess County, New York, Department of Health and former president of the National Association of County and City Health Officials, says, "Most public health professionals do not look at the bioterrorism money to solve all our social ills, but to expand our 'dual-use,' which means surveillance and response functions of communicable diseases." But as the Government Accountability Office recently confirmed, others worry that the massive shift of resources into traditional emergency response areas such as fire departments and law enforcement will detract from the pressing needs of the medical and public health sectors and impair their ability to detect and respond to bioterrorism. A Council of State and Territorial Epidemiologists report recommended that "dual use of terrorism and emergency preparedness epidemiology resources should be substantially expanded to realign functional roles and build overall capacity of state health departments to prepare for and respond to terrorism, infectious disease outbreaks, and other public health threats and emergencies."

Many in general government feared that a narrow focus on health as an adjunct to national defense could undermine health agencies' broader mission to provide a variety of services not necessarily tied to bioterrorism and emergency preparedness. The economic recessions that in some states had begun before 9/11 strained state budgets and forced spending reductions for many state functions, including health. As time passed, the need to respond to the events of late 2001 seemed less urgent and population health preparedness became just one of a number of different budget priorities that legislators had to consider in tough fiscal times. The budgetary problems were magnified by the federal mandate in late 2002 to institute a major smallpox inoculation campaign.

The attempt to codify and reformulate state public health laws with the draft Model State Emergency Health Powers Act, together with what some criticized as the poor federal handling of the anthrax episode and smallpox inoculation campaign, served to stimulate a broad discussion of the new obligations and responsibilities of health authorities. Some worried that an emphasis on surveillance techniques and disease reporting, though long a part of public health management, might undermine public trust in the system as a whole if seen as an infringement on personal liberties. In the aftermath of September 11, the clash of conflicting values—setting the rights of individuals against the perceived need for greater bioterrorism preparedness—has heightened the sense of disorder for officials already dealing with the swift and radical transformation of their jobs.

Protecting the CDC's Accomplishments Against New Priorities

The federal government, through the CDC, has accomplished a great deal in its efforts to improve emergency response and bioterrorism preparedness. Notably, in addition to aiding individual states and cities, it has expanded the National Laboratory Response Network, increased the Strategic National Stockpile of pharmaceuticals and medical supplies and ensured their delivery to any place in the United States within twelve hours, and developed new technologies for more effective systems of surveillance and data sharing. But, as Joseph Henderson puts it, "The key concern today is to assure that federal, state, and government leaders and elected officials don't sacrifice the ground gained since September 11 due to new priorities and shifting political interests. Significant resources are in place to support broad-based public health including public health readiness. One cannot exist without the other. A solid public health system strives to reduce/eliminate illness, injury, and death every day but especially when a catastrophic event occurs such as bioterrorism or SARS."

Maintaining the public health infrastructure is probably the single most important means of preparing the nation for the myriad unpredictable crises arising from naturally occurring epidemics as well as from terrorist attacks. Without a strong permanent infrastructure, the best emergency planning will be inadequate. The financial difficulties of the various states, combined with the federal government's shift in focus from bioterrorism and terrorism in general to smallpox and the war in Iraq in particular, have lessened the chance of achieving what had seemed likely immediately after 9/11: enhancement of the system of services that are essential to improve national bioterrorism preparedness and to address the overall health needs of the American people.

Public Health
Along the Border

Jim Atkinson

The rural settlements along the U.S.–Mexico border are among the sickest places in Texas, according to Jim Atkinson, the author of the following article. Mostly populated by poor Mexican Americans, the settlements (colonias in Spanish) consist of jerry-built houses or trailers without adequate heating or proper septic systems. The residents are exposed to environmental pollution that floats over the border from factories in Mexico or from pesticides from nearby farms. Diabetes, tuberculosis, hepatitis B, and hypertension are common diseases that go undertreated. The colonias present a challenge for government as well as for the public and health professionals.

The lack of insurance among residents of the colonias is a major hindrance to medical care. As Atkinson reports, few health-care corporations will open clinics where most of the population is uninsured and unable to pay for services. Lacking adequate care in Texas, many people cross the border to buy medications on the street. If something is not done soon to cure the colonias the diseases they breed could easily infect other parts of the region.

These impoverished settlements along the Mexican border are certifiably the sickest places in Texas. But not for the reasons you think.

"That looks like a cesspool," says Leticia Paez, the director of an El Paso non-profit public health care organization, as she eases her car around a corner in the east El Paso County colonia known as Las Pompas. Sure enough, behind a mobile home is an expanse of standing water that seems to be leaking from a septic tank.

As we drive by it, we see something else: a beautiful array of flowers on the porch of the trailer next door.

The colonias are like that. The pride of ownership is apparent and, if you can ignore the dust and the flies and the stray animals, there is something oddly romantic about these ramshackle settlements. For better or worse, this is how the nation was settled—by poor, humble people daring to build whatever they could afford on small slips of desolate land bought on credit.

The Mexican Americans who inhabit these odd little rural settlements along the border—which now number 1,500 and are home to 400,000 citizens (most of them, contrary to popular belief, legal)—are poor and uneducated and work in agricultural industries or in low-wage service-industry jobs. They wind up here because they want to own their own homes but can't afford anything more than a plot of raw land in unzoned regions of border counties. Here, they can put a few dollars down and then pay on average $225 a month to a developer for the privilege of either building their homes with discarded or stolen construction materials or buying a used trailer. Their deal with the developer may or may not include water and sewage hookups.

A Breeding Ground for Disease

What they also get for their money is one of the worst breeding grounds for disease in America. Around every corner, it seems, new health hazards pop up like cardboard monsters in a fun house. Many of the makeshift homes can be brutally cold in the winter. Unburied septic tanks sit worrisomely close to the large drums of purchased drinking water in yards landscaped only with varying shades and consistencies of dust, which may be laced with pesticides from nearby farms. A faint scent of pollution is in the air; some of it probably comes from the maquiladoras [assembly plants] across the border in Juarez, but much of it is locally generated by people who burn their trash, which sometimes includes dead animals.

What you don't see is as worrisome as what you do. The air and water here are thick with microbes. Tuberculosis [TB], hepatitis A, and Helicobacter pylori (the bug responsible for many stomach ulcers) all travel freely across the border and are more prevalent here than in other parts of the state. Add to that the near plague of diabetes and hypertension among Hispanic adults and the substance abuse and depression that come with living in such oppressive poverty, and it's no wonder that some of these colonias are among the sickest places in Texas—maybe even in the nation.

A Lack of Health-Care Facilities

The conventional wisdom is that the colonias are sick because they lack safe drinking water and adequate sewage facilities. Twenty years ago that was probably true. But in the past few years, amazing progress has been made in solving those problems, the direct result of some $600 million in federal and state expenditures. And while some health problems still come from poor water and sewage, the Texas Department of Health now says that only an estimated 10 to 15 percent of colonia households are not hooked up to potable drinking water, and most of them are able to buy suitable water. And almost all residents are either connected to a public sewer system or have septic tanks (though the Department of Health would not swear by the viability of many of those tanks or their drain fields).

The real problem in the colonias these days is something you might not notice when you first drive through: the staggering lack of health care facilities. Many more colonia settlers have greater access to water and sewage facilities than they do to health insurance or hospitals; the sickest places in Texas are that way, in part, because they don't have enough doctors and nurses. According to the Department of Health, 64 percent of colonia households have no private health coverage; another 20 percent have only partial coverage. And while about 30 percent of colonia residents get Medicaid, that still leaves a lot of people without any health coverage.

Since health care, perversely, tends to follow money rather than sickness, it should come as no surprise that all but 2 of 43 border counties have been judged "medically underserved" or that a study by the comptrollers office found that 22 community clinics along the border had to handle a staggering 700,000 medical and dental visits by 200,000 patients during a recent year. Public hospitals with emergency rooms or specialty services are often miles away; emergency medical service is a pipe dream. Paez, who is the director of Kellogg Community Partnership, an organization that runs four clinics that provide health care to several colonias, could name only seven clinics that serve the 72,000 people who live in El Paso County's 214 colonias. "Schools can be tied in to economic development," she explained. "That's why you'll see big, shiny schools around some of the colonias. But health care is just not part of that equation because it basically serves people with little economic influence: the elderly and the poor." That's true—no city ever sold a corporate relocation based on the health services provided to its poor neighborhoods.

But the colonias' health care deficit also has to do with a certain assumption that has always been made about health and the poor: That, all things considered, the residents would just as soon live in squalor and ill health, and that even if you made facilities and information available, they wouldn't avail themselves of them. This has always been especially presumed of the residents of colonias, given their insistence on an independent and somewhat isolated rural lifestyle. "I think there is an unfair presumption in that direction," says Dr. Janet Gildea, a nun who runs the Clinica Guadalupana, which serves half a dozen colonias near the small town of Horizon City, in east El Paso County. "But until we opened six years ago, no one was coming to these people and saying, 'We want you healthy.' I've found that if you take the time, the patients will do what they need to do. The much bigger problem is whether they can pay for it." Medicaid or the State Children's Health Insurance Program (SCHIP) covers some of the children who come to the clinic. But most of the adults are classified as "self pay," meaning they are uninsured and can pay only a nominal fee of $10 or so. The cruel irony is that many of them don't qualify for public coverage (adult Medicaid) because they have jobs and some income—but not enough, of course, to afford private insurance.

But that fact doesn't seem to be keeping them away from the doctor's office. On a recent Wednesday morning, Gildea's waiting room at the clinic—a rambling, freshly painted flame house—was swamped with remarkably cheerful people who seemed glad to have any clinic. Mothers were there to have their kids treated for skin, eye, and stomach infections that are common in the colonias, or to have their own diabetes or hypertension monitored. Patients were being counseled on critical public health issues such as antibiotic abuse, the tendency of Mexican immigrants to head back across the border for a cheap shot of the drugs whenever they feel ill—a habit that many doctors believe has contributed to the development of drug-resistant strains of infections such as tuberculosis.

Getting Health Care to the People

Gloria Morales, who does clerical work for Gildea, is a dramatic example of what a difference the presence of health care facilities can make. Five years ago, before she began working for the clinic, Morales would cross the border to "get a shot of antibiotics anytime I felt sick with anything. Only I, wouldn't always work. So I finally came here, and Dr. Gildea found out I have diabetes. Now I try to find and educate people who are like I was." Much as a police patrol car can help bring order and civility to a community by its mere presence, a clinic and a doctor can raise the level of public health just by being there. But it takes a certain critical mass to begin to make real progress. Gildea says that her clinic can handle checkups and screenings and education, but if she has to make a special referral, she often has trouble placing an uninsured patient. As the only clinic in an area with a potential patient base of 10,000, she worries that "at any time, something like cholera could break out, and then what would we do?"

How best to get a Clinica Guadalupana on every corner? One school of thought insists that it's better to relocate these settlers closer to health services. "We are better served if we use the money we spend on water to give them housing vouchers to pay for regulated housing in the city," says state senator Eliot Shapleigh, an El Paso Democrat whose territory includes a number of colonias. "The colonias are a symptom, not the problem. The problem is poverty."

Fair enough. But if some of the colonias continue to be the sickest places in Texas, many of them have matured into reasonably safe and healthy places, and you'd hate to discourage these scrappy settlers just when they've begun to stand on their own. Besides, most of these settlements, feeble as they are, haven't displayed the slightest willingness to die. So how does one get more health care to come to them, without just throwing more money at completely subsidized clinics or treatment? Something that could help immediately to encourage residents to take better care of themselves is some form of low-cost, partly subsidized health coverage. I'm thinking along the lines of one big HMO [health maintenance organization] for the colonias. Residents would receive a voucher from the State of Texas, add to it what they could, and purchase their own health insurance—somewhat like the SCHIP for children. This plan has several virtues. First, and most obviously, it would improve treatment options. But it would also attract more medical services closer to the colonias because it would represent the money that such services always follow. Most important, it would play to the colonia residents' greatest strength: their insistence on self-determination. Many of the patients at the Clinica Guadalupana may be able to afford only $10 a visit, but most of them pay it proudly, and I have no doubt they would pay a modest insurance premium as well.

Finally, this isn't just a matter of improving the health care of a uniquely vulnerable population. It's also a matter of regulating what could become a public health threat to any or all of us, which is why we should use state tax dollars to subsidize the insurance. Even though the colonias seem isolated, their health can affect yours. Microbes are built for long-distance travel, and all it takes is one carrier to pass along drug-resistant TB. As Paez says, "In public health, if you don't pay now, you always pay later."

An Outbreak of SARS in Toronto Illustrates Ways to Fight a Future Epidemic

Susan Poutanen

In 2002 and 2003 the city of Toronto, Canada, experienced an outbreak of SARS (severe acute respiratory syndrome) a highly contagious disease characterized by fever, headache, and body aches, followed by a dry cough that may lead to great difficulty in breathing. The movement of SARS around the world was a classic example of pandemic disease. It appeared in November 2002 in China and soon spread to Hong Kong. From Hong Kong it spread via air travelers to east Asia, North America, and Europe and the rest of the world.

Public health officials around the world imposed strict control measures, including prohibitions on travel to and from affected countries as well as quarantines of hospitals and other places where persons were found to be infected. By June 2003 the spread of SARS had been controlled to the point where restrictions were eased. The following article describes the methods used by the Canadian city to address the crisis. Author Susan Poutanen, a microbiologist at the Toronto Medical Laboratories and Mount Sinai Hospital Department of Microbiology, writes that lessons learned about communications, deployment of staff, ethics versus the needs of researchers, and morale provide vital guidelines for dealing with future pandemics.

Whether it be a lab accident, release of a biologic weapon into the community, the next flu pandemic, or the next SARS (severe acute respiratory syndrome) outbreak, clinical laboratories must be prepared for possible biohazard and bioterror emergencies.

Susan Poutanen, "Do Your Biohazard, Bioterror and Emergency Planning Now," *Medical Laboratory Observer*, vol. 39, February 2007, p. 38. © 2007 Nelson Publishing Inc. All rights reserved. Reproduced by permission.

Clinical laboratories in Toronto [Canada] faced such an emergency during the 2002–2003 SARS outbreak that affected 26 countries and was associated with 8,096 cases and 774 deaths worldwide. In Canada, 251 cases and 43 deaths were reported—the majority of which were hospital-acquired in various Toronto hospitals. Hospital-based labs were mostly affected; and while some had emergency plans, many only had drafts or no plans. All were faced with real-time decision making, adapting daily to the outbreak as it unfolded throughout the city. In the end, the outbreak was controlled and the majority of clinical laboratories have since reviewed their practices and implemented changes based on the many lessons learned from this experience. The impact that the SARS outbreak had on our laboratory and how we responded are presented here with a summary of what we did well and what we could have done better, and recommendations for laboratory biohazard or bioterror emergency planning and preparedness.

Responding to the Outbreak

In Canada, all hospitals and hospital-affiliated laboratories are government-funded. Our laboratory is an academic containment level-2 microbiology service shared between two large academic hospitals. At the time of the SARS outbreak, we had two sites—one housed within an academic hospital and one in an offsite building. We serve a total of nine Ontario hospitals with approximately 5,000 beds and five non-hospital clients. Approximately 40,000 specimens are processed per month.

On March 13, 2003, the World Health Organization (WHO) released an e-mail alert regarding a severe respiratory syndrome in Hong Kong and Vietnam. The following day, we became aware of patients with possible SARS in two of our client hospitals including the base hospital in which one of our sites was located. A local press release was issued, and teleconferences were immediately set up with the WHO, Health Canada, and Greater Toronto Area infectious-disease physicians and microbiologists. A description of the first patients was placed on ProMED-mail [global electronic reporting system for outbreaks of diseases and toxin] in an attempt to alert the worldwide medical community as quickly as possible.

Intense contact tracing of the initial cluster of cases soon revealed that three to four generations of spread had already occurred in Toronto. The exact numbers and extent of the outbreak were not immediately obvious, and headlines declared the outbreak was "out of control." The index hospital in which the initial cluster of cases was admitted was forced to close, with all new admissions deferred and all elective patients discharged. All hospitals, including laboratories contained within hospital buildings, were put under a provincial "Code Orange" with mandatory directives to use . . . respirators at all times. SARS units were created, and all healthcare workers were instructed to use . . . respirators with droplet and contact precautions on these wards.

Healthy hygiene was advocated including not coming to work sick, covering a cough, washing hands, and not touching noses and mouths. Hospitals were asked to run only essential services, and only essential hospital workers were allowed to work at only one hospital site. Visitors were limited, and entry and exit points from all hospital buildings were secured. All persons entering the hospitals were screened for symptoms compatible with SARS. Daily updates from public-health officials shared the total number of cases and deaths related to the outbreak, and daily updates of provincial hospital directives were released regularly to all hospital administrators.

After three months, the outbreak was declared ended, and Toronto was taken off the WHO SARS list, only to be put back on it within a week after unrecognized cases were discovered. Another month passed before the second wave of the Toronto outbreak was controlled, and the city was again taken off the WHO SARS list.

Challenges to Laboratories

Our laboratory, primarily our hospital-based site, was faced with many challenges as the SARS outbreak unfolded.

Challenge 1: Our laboratory and the hospital within which we were housed did not have an outbreak-preparedness plan. Forced to make real-time decisions and policies on a daily basis, we had to determine how to communicate daily protocol changes in an efficient way. The lack of a single reliable communications system for all heathcare workers required that updates be sent via e-mail, websites, and faxes. Daily televised provincial public-health updates and daily teleconferences with physicians from SARS-affected hospitals were broadcast publicly. Within the laboratory, electronic messages and stand-up meetings were used.

Challenge 2: How to handle specimens when dealing with an unknown pathogen with an unknown mode and extent of transmissibility in an open-concept laboratory was particularly demanding for all labs. . . .

Challenge 3: Handling operations with decreased staff numbers was another Herculean task. Staff numbers dropped due to one of many possibilities: being sick, being on quarantine or home isolation, being redeployed within the hospital (e.g., to screen incoming healthcare workers), or being deemed a non-essential worker. Daily updates to our laboratory bench schedule were required, and we had to reprioritize which lab tests could be completed, keeping in mind those tests that were in increased demand such as respiratory-pathogen testing. The value of cross-trained staff was evident in helping to reschedule benches at the last minute.

Challenge 4: Responding to the demand from front-line clinicians and epidemiologists for a diagnostic test was also problematic. . . .

Challenge 5: Autopsies were sought by many in an attempt to better understand SARS, but many pathologists refused to complete them, many families refused to have them performed, and coordination with obtaining appropriate specimens was not easy. The province elected to have all suspected SARS deaths reviewed by the coroner with mandated autopsies as appropriate. All autopsies were completed in a centralized location with one central point-person from our microbiology lab and one from our associated pathology lab to coordinate specimen handling and transportation. . . .

Challenge 6: Following metrics throughout the outbreak also proved to be difficult. . . .

Challenge 7: Finally, working in an environment of fear for weeks on end proved to be formidable. Witnessing friends and colleagues get sick, and hearing daily reports of death counts was disheartening for staff. Open communication and encouragement to share emotions with one another was an important coping mechanism.

The Report Card on Dealing with SARS

In retrospect, we did many things well to cope with the SARS outbreak. For example, having routinely scheduled daily provincial televised updates was an excellent communication strategy. . . . Forming a collaborative laboratory working-group proved useful to enable validation of novel diagnostic tests. Centralizing autopsies, and coordinating responsible microbiology and pathology laboratory personnel was key to obtaining appropriate autopsy specimens. Having SARS-specific ethics-board reviews was critical in getting research proposals appraised in a timely fashion. Finally, having an open-communication policy was important for staff as a coping strategy.

While many things worked for us during the SARS outbreak, we could have done many things better. For example, using paper requisition and results proved tedious and prevented easy capture of data regarding the use of novel diagnostics. Delays in collating data impaired real-time understanding of the outbreak and impeded research progress. Applying to multiple research-ethics review boards was very time-consuming and inefficient. Finally, the lack of readily updateable metrics prevented the capture of the true impact of the outbreak on our laboratory.

Caring for Wounded War Veterans Will Strain the Nation's Public Health System

Nancy Shute, Elizabeth Querna, and Susan Brink et al.

The medical needs of soldiers wounded in the war in Iraq present special problems for the nation's military hospitals and public health-care systems. Unlike veterans of previous wars, current soldiers are surviving traumatic amputations and head wounds due to the protective body armor they wear and the emergency medical treatment they receive. Once they return home, however, the most severely wounded soldiers may need lifetime care or months of expensive rehabilitation.

Many observers of the health needs of veterans doubt there is enough money to provide this level of extreme care either through the Veterans Administration [VA] or through private health insurers. The VA, which traditionally provides two years of free health care to veterans, may be unable to continue to do so in the face of rising demand. They will have to decide who receives an artificial leg or reconstructive facial surgery. Veterans who choose to work with doctors, hospitals, and rehab facilities outside the VA face huge medical bills that they may or may not be able to pay. Those who cannot return to work due to physical or medical disabilities place pressures on the social services of their communities. The looming health-care crisis facing the war wounded is the topic of the following article.

"**M**om, is that you? I'm alive."

When Pat Coleman heard those words in a midnight phone call, she knew her son had been wounded in Iraq.

David Coleman, a 20-year-old Marine lance corporal, was calling home on a satellite phone to Butte, Mont., from a hospital in Baghdad [Iraq]. He didn't know how badly he was injured. Only later would he learn that he'd nearly bled to death, that the improvised explosive device [IED] that ripped open his armored humvee on September 23 had shattered both his legs, and that he had only a fifty-fifty shot at not having his right leg amputated. At that point, the young marine knew only that he was about to be evacuated to the Landstuhl Regional Medical Center in Germany and that everyone said if you made it to Landstuhl, you were going to be OK.

"I remember everything, like a movie," Coleman said from his bed at Landstuhl four days later, his eyes wide and black from anesthesia three hours after surgery to clean his wounds. "Boom! There was dust. There was smoke. People were screaming, 'I'm hit! I'm hit!'" Blood was pouring out of his boot. Coleman remembers hearing someone say, "He's got 10 minutes before the shock kills him" and realizing that the guy was talking about him. "There was blood everywhere." Less wounded buddies carried Coleman to another humvee for the drive to a medevac helicopter and a short flight to a forward surgical team. Surgeons stopped the bleeding; then Coleman was ferried to a combat support hospital at Asad Airfield, where doctors performed emergency surgery to stabilize his legs. After spending the night in Baghdad, Coleman was strapped to a litter and loaded onto a C-141 transport plane to Germany. He arrived barely 36 hours after the IED shredded his humvee and had been in Iraq just 10 days. "I'm the first soldier from Montana to be injured," he said, with a dazed smile. "I wanted to be a part of Marine Corps history. And now I am."

Better Stats

Landstuhl is the first step in the long journey home for David Coleman and the nearly 9,500 other soldiers who have been wounded in Iraq and Afghanistan. Unbeknown to them, they are part of a great experiment in military medicine. Soldiers today are far more likely to survive battle than in any other war in American history. In World War II, 1 in 3 casualties died. Even in the relatively bloodless 1991 Gulf War, 147 were killed in battle, 467 wounded in action. In Iraq and Afghanistan, however, 98 percent of those wounded have survived. "Mortality is down about 22 percent" compared with the first Gulf War, says Dale Smith, chairman of medical history at the Uniformed Services University of the Health Sciences. He credits better protection for soldiers, as well as improved medical care. "It's phenomenal progress, at phenomenal expense."

As more soldiers come home with physical injuries and mental health problems, it becomes increasingly clear that survival has other, greater costs. The nation's healthcare system for veterans is already overburdened, and federal officials and veterans groups fear the country won't fulfill its promise to care for its wounded soldiers for the rest of their lives.

During the Vietnam War, it could take a wounded soldier a month to make it home for treatment. Iraq is different, partly because it's an urban battlefield and partly because the military has radically retooled its system of treatment and evacuation. "We have to provide fast, flexible medical care," says Lt. Col. Slobodan Jazarevic, a vascular surgeon at Landstuhl who is returning to Iraq to head the 44th Medical Command. "There are no lines of battle. The battle is fought everywhere."

Badly wounded patients like Coleman are quickly flown to Landstuhl and spend three to five days there before being shipped to the States. The very ill move even faster. "The biggest change in military medicine in the past 10 years has been the CCATs [critical care air transports]—flying ICUs [intensive care units]," says Air Force Col. Kory Cornum, an orthopedic surgeon who commands the 86th Medical Squadron at

Landstuhl. Cornum recently operated on a patient who was in the intensive care unit at Walter Reed Army Medical Center in Washington, D.C., just 36 hours after being badly wounded in Iraq. "Our country's the only country that can do that," Cornum says. "Not the only country that can but the only country that will."

At Landstuhl, a hospital that had become a snoozy Cold War relic is back in full war mode; more than 20,000 patients have arrived from Iraq and Afghanistan since the wars began. After the battle in Fallujah began, on November 8, the hospital took in 455 patients in a week. When the call goes out on the hospital PA [public address] system that a plane from downrange is "wheels down" at nearby Ramstein Air Base, staff members start lining up gurneys outside the emergency room door. The critically ill arrive first, by ambulance; their CCAT teams wheel them directly to intensive care or an operating room.

24-7

More-stable patients like Coleman are carried off buses on litters. Those with bad backs and other less pressing health problems—the "disease nonbattle injury" cases, which make up the bulk of troop loss in any war, far more than from enemy fire—walk off the bus themselves and are handed a list of their doctor appointments and a phone card so they can call home. The traffic is choreographed in the Deployed Warrior Medical Management Center, a fancy name for a handful of modular offices in the parking lot outside the ER [emergency room]. There, doctors, nurses, and dispatchers work 24-7, monitoring an online database where their counterparts in the Middle East list the incoming wounded—multiple trauma from a vehicle rollover, abdominal pain, amputations. Says Capt. Monabell Vamvas, a triage nurse and reservist from Glendale, Calif.: "I know every person on that flight."

If the rapid evacuations are one of the big medical success stories of this war, another is improved body armor, which physicians credit with much of the reduced death rate. Flak jackets have been used for decades, but even in the 1991 Gulf War, they weren't capable of stopping high-velocity rifle rounds. Now they do. "It is also different because soldiers wear it," says Army Col. David Burris, a trauma surgeon and interim chairman of surgery at the Uniformed Services University of the Health Sciences. "It's thrilling, I'd much rather prevent an injury than fix it."

But the vests don't prevent all injuries. Because arms and legs aren't protected, extremity injuries like Coleman's now account for some 70 percent of battlefield wounds. Surgeons say the damage is comparable to a catastrophic machinery accident back home. At least 152 soldiers have had limbs amputated; the number of traumatic brain injuries is also up. But it's as yet impossible to tell if those injury rates have increased, partly because the number of survivors has risen, skewing the statistics, and because the Army is compiling its trauma registry from paper records. One wounded soldier could have records at three or four places in Iraq and could arrive at Landstuhl with medical records and X-rays on his Army blanket or with no records at all.

Simple Solutions

Surgeons say the use of new fast-clot bandages and better tourniquets and access to fresh whole blood are helping to keep severely wounded patients from bleeding to death. The fact that trauma teams trained together at civilian trauma centers back home helps, too, according to Col. John Holcomb, commander of the Army Institute of Surgical Research. But sometimes even a simple solution can help. Soldiers were suffering devastating eye injuries from shrapnel, but doctors realized such injuries could be prevented if the soldiers wore sunglasses with shatterproof polycarbonate lenses, such as

WileyXs. "Most of the injuries were from people who got sweaty and took their glasses off for one second," says James Burden, one of four ophthalmologists at Landstuhl. Once the Army distributed posters with gruesome injury photos, the sunglasses stayed on. Says Burden: "We've seen injuries drop dramatically."

The patients are also changing battlefield medicine. Forty percent of the troops in Iraq are National Guard and Reserve, who are older than active-duty soldiers and more likely to have heart problems or back trouble. "A fair number of reservists and National Guard were activated with cataracts," says Burden. "Once they go into theater with the bright sunshine, they started complaining of problems. We fix them up and send them back."

For seriously wounded soldiers like Coleman, the next step on the journey home is a military hospital stateside. Because he's a marine, Coleman wound up in the National Naval Medical Center in Bethesda, Md. His parents took unpaid leave from their jobs to be at his bedside. Coleman spent the fall undergoing surgery and fighting off a staph infection, making the slow progression from hospital bed to wheelchair to, finally, a walker. "I can wiggle my toes!" he exclaimed last week, two months after shrapnel from the IED tore into his legs. His right leg is no longer in peril. His new calf, which surgeons built out of muscle grafts from his abdomen and skin grafts from his flank, flexes as if it had always been there. But he still has a long way to go; at least one more surgery for bone and nerve grafts, then lengthy physical therapy. On his bedside table, on top of his laptop, lies an application for veterans' disability benefits. "I'm torn right now," he says of the decision ahead—to try to stay in the Marine Corps or seek a medical discharge and use his benefits to go to film school. "If I can do the job I came into the Marine Corps to do, then I want to go back. I'll have to see what they say."

The path from military medicine to the Department of Veterans Affairs [VA] which is charged with providing care to the nation's 24.7 million veterans, is, all too often, no simple stroll down easy street. The Defense Department and the VA have separate medical systems and separate medical boards that determine soldiers' eligibility for benefits. Efforts are underway to remove some of the roadblocks. The VA now has representatives at 136 military installations, including Landstuhl and Bethesda. The Pentagon has a new program, the Disabled Soldier Support System, with 10 counselors around the country. The VA and the Pentagon are working on a two-way electronic medical records system, which VA Secretary Anthony Principi says will be in place next year. Since 1998, the departments also have been trying to establish one-stop medical exams that would work for both military discharge and veterans benefits. Just this month, the Government Accountability Office reported that four of eight single-exam programs touted by the VA didn't exist and that the military often diverted funds for the project to healthcare for active-duty soldiers.

Returnees from Iraq and Afghanistan are guaranteed two years' free healthcare by the VA. Veterans groups give the VA high marks for quality of care; over the past decade it has pioneered patient-safety programs like computerized prescription entry, considered vital for reducing medical errors. But the system faces increased demand. Enrollment has risen from 4.8 million to 7.6 million since 2001. "The VA is not ready for an influx of new veterans," says Rep. Lane Evans, ranking Democrat on the House Veterans Affairs Committee. "It is managing by rationing healthcare services."

Last year, in an effort to stretch the dollars, the VA eliminated healthcare benefits for vets who make more than about $30,000 a year; the agency has also proposed increasing user fees. And although the VA has cut the wait for an initial primary-care visit down to 30 days for most patients, it can take months to see an eye doctor or oncologist. "Often the appointment to see a specialist is 10 months to a year," says Cathy Wiblemo, deputy director for healthcare for the American Legion. Principi says it may take six months to see an orthopedist for a hip replacement, "but I'm not sure that's that much different than the private sector."

When his long convalescence is over, David Coleman isn't sure where he will be headed. But . . . he got some great news: The Marine Corps decided he'd be better off recuperating at home in Montana for 30 days before his next surgery. As soon as the paperwork is done, Coleman will be headed for the airport. He says: "I will be home for Thanksgiving."

Climate Change Is Affecting the World's Health in a Multitude of Ways

World Health Organization

The gradual warming of the Earth's climate is largely attributed to emissions produced by industrialized societies such as the United States. Yet all societies, industrialized, industrializing, and agricultural, are experiencing the effects of the change in a multitude of ways. These include altered growing seasons, the rise of sea levels and flooding of lowlands, the spread of diseases such as malaria, and deaths caused by extremes in temperature.

The following summary prepared by the World Health Organization (WHO) describes the relationship between climate change and human health. The report concludes that it may take decades for the poorest nations to recover from epidemics or natural disasters caused by climate change. Lacking basic public health-care systems the poor nations of the world will be hard-pressed to help their people survive outbreaks of disease, deal with natural disasters, or even feed themselves in times of drought.

In 1969, the Apollo moon shot provided extraordinary photographs of this planet, suspended in space. This transformed how we thought about the biosphere and its limits.

Our increasing understanding of climate change is transforming how we view the boundaries and determinants of human health. While our personal health may seem to relate mostly to prudent behaviour, heredity, occupation, local environmental exposures, and health-care access, sustained population health requires the life-supporting "services" of the bio-

World Health Organization, "Climate Change and Human Health—Risks and Responses," 2003. © Copyright World Health Organization (WHO). Reproduced by permission.

sphere. Populations of all animal species depend on supplies of food and water, freedom from excess infectious disease, and the physical safety and comfort conferred by climatic stability. The world's climate system is fundamental to this life-support.

Humans Are Responsible for Warming the Planet

Today, humankind's activities are altering the world's climate. We are increasing the atmospheric concentration of energy-trapping gases, thereby amplifying the natural "greenhouse effect" that makes the Earth habitable. These greenhouse gases (GHGs) comprise, principally, carbon dioxide (mostly from fossil fuel combustion and forest burning), plus other heat-trapping gases such as methane (from irrigated agriculture, animal husbandry and oil extraction), nitrous oxide and various human-made halocarbons.

In its Third Assessment Report (2001), the UN's [United Nations'] Intergovernmental Panel on Climate Change (IPCC) stated: "There is new and stronger evidence that most of the warming observed over the last 50 years is attributable to human activities."

During the twentieth century, world average surface temperature increased by approximately 0.6°C, and approximately two-thirds of that warming has occurred since 1975. Climatologists forecast further warming, along with changes in precipitation and climatic variability, during the coming century and beyond. Their forecasts are based on increasingly sophisticated global climate models, applied to plausible future scenarios of global greenhouse gas emissions that take into account alternative trajectories for demographic, economic and technological changes and evolving patterns of governance.

The global scale of climate change differs fundamentally from the many other familiar environmental concerns that refer to localised toxicological or microbiological hazards. Indeed, climate change signifies that, today, we are altering

Earth's biophysical and ecological systems at the planetary scale—as is also evidenced by stratospheric ozone depletion, accelerating biodiversity losses, stresses on terrestrial and marine food-producing systems, depletion of freshwater supplies, and the global dissemination of persistent organic pollutants.

Human societies have had long experience of naturally-occurring climatic vicissitudes [changes]. The ancient Egyptians, Mesopotamians, Mayans, and European populations (during the four centuries of the Little Ice Age) were all affected by nature's great climatic cycles. More acutely, disasters and disease outbreaks have occurred often in response to the extremes of regional climatic cycles such as the El Niño Southern Oscillation (ENSO) cycle.

The IPCC (2001) has estimated that the global average temperature will rise by several degrees centigrade during this century. There is unavoidable uncertainty in this estimate, since the intricacies of the climate system are not fully understood, and humankind's developmental future cannot be foretold with certainty.

World temperature has increased by around 0.4°C since the 1970s, and now exceeds the upper limit of natural (historical) variability. Climatologists assess that most of that recent increase is due to human influence.

Impacts on Human Health

Change in world climate would influence the functioning of many ecosystems and their member species. Likewise, there would be impacts on human health. Some of these health impacts would be beneficial. For example, milder winters would reduce the seasonal winter-time peak in deaths that occurs in temperate countries, while in currently hot regions a further increase in temperatures might reduce the viability of disease-transmitting mosquito populations. Overall, however, scientists consider that most of the health impacts of climate change would be adverse.

Climatic changes over recent decades have probably already affected some health outcomes. Indeed, the World Health Organisation [WHO], estimated, in its "World Health Report 2002", that climate change was estimated to be responsible in 2000 for approximately 2.4% of worldwide diarrhoea, and 6% of malaria in some middle-income countries. However, small changes, against a noisy background of ongoing changes in other causal factors, are hard to identify. Once spotted, causal attribution is strengthened if there are similar observations in different population settings.

The first detectable changes in human health may well be alterations in the geographic range (latitude and altitude) and seasonality of certain infectious diseases—including vector-borne infections such as malaria and dengue fever, and food-borne infections (e.g. salmonellosis) which peak in the warmer months. Warmer average temperatures combined with increased climatic variability would alter the pattern of exposure to thermal extremes and resultant health impacts, in both summer and winter. By contrast, the public health consequences of the disturbance of natural and managed food-producing ecosystems, rising sea-levels and population displacement for reasons of physical hazard, land loss, economic disruption and civil strife, may not become evident for up to several decades.

Unprecedentedly, today, the world population is encountering unfamiliar human-induced changes in the lower and middle atmospheres and world-wide depletion of various other natural systems (e.g. soil fertility, aquifers, ocean fisheries, and biodiversity in general). Beyond the early recognition that such changes would affect economic activities, infrastructure and managed ecosystems, there is now recognition that global climate change poses risks to human population health.

This topic is emerging as a major theme in population health research, social policy development, and advocacy. Indeed, consideration of global climatic-environmental hazards to human health will become a central role in the sustainability transition debate.

Chronology

312 B.C.
The Romans build the first aqueduct to carry clean water from distant springs and streams to the city of Rome.

A.D. 370
St. Basil builds the first hospital in the Roman Empire in Caesarea. It includes an isolation ward for lepers and buildings for the poor, elderly, and sick.

549
Byzantine emperor Justinian I rules that people arriving in Constantinople from regions infected with bubonic plague should be hindered in their movements and isolated from the rest of the population.

600s
The imperial government of China establishes a policy to hold sailors and travelers who arrive in Chinese ports carrying the plague.

1300s
Bethlem Royal Hospital (Bedlam) in London, initially founded to care for the sick poor and homeless, admits the insane.

1348
The appearance of bubonic plague in Europe prompts the government of the Venetian city-state to establish the world's first organized system of quarantine. The city council has the power to detain ships and their cargoes, crews, and passengers offshore for forty days.

1647
Mindful of the dangers of epidemics the government of the Massachusetts Bay Colony requires all ships arriving in the port of Boston to pause in the harbor or risk a fine. By the 1700s all the major towns and cities along the eastern seaboard have quarantine laws.

1798

The Marine Hospital Service is established in the United States to care for sick seamen in American ports. It evolves into the Public Health Service (PHS).

1832

New York City experiences its first outbreak of cholera. More than three thousand New Yorkers, mainly slum dwellers, die during a two-month period.

1854

In London, Dr. John Snow confirms his theory that cholera is spread through contaminated water. He persuades city officials to remove the handle of the water pump in the stricken neighborhood and in a few days the epidemic subsides.

1865

Construction of London's sewer system is completed. Over thirteen hundred miles of pipes carry sewage away from the city for release into the Thames.

1866

The Metropolitan Board of Health is established in New York City and oversees public health rules for the city.

1878

The National Quarantine Act grants authority for quarantine (once under the control of the states) to the Marine Hospital Service.

1893

Public health nursing begins with the founding of the Henry Street Settlement in New York City. Its founder, Lillian Wald, coins the term "public health nurse."

1906

Congress passes the Pure Food and Drug Act thereby authorizing the government to monitor the purity of food and the safety of drugs.

1907

Mary Mallon is arrested for being a carrier of typhoid fever and is placed in isolation on an island in New York City. Public health officials keep her there for the rest of her life to protect the city populace.

1915

U.S. Public Health Service surgeon and epidemiologist Joseph Goldberger concludes that a high-carbohydrate, high fat, and no-protein diet causes pellagra, a disease prevalent in the southern states. The widespread poverty of the Great Depression leads to policy changes that eradicated pellagra from the United States and other developed countries.

1918–1919

A worldwide influenza epidemic strikes in the United States and kills six hundred thousand. It illustrates the nation's lack of a unified and prepared federal and regional public health system.

1946

The Communicable Disease Center is established. It is the forerunner of the Centers for Disease Control and Prevention (CDC).

1948

Killer smog in Donora, Pennsylvania kills twenty and hospitalizes over seven thousand and leads to the Clean Air Act of 1970.

1953

The Department of Health, Education, and Welfare (HEW) is created by President Dwight D. Eisenhower.

1954

Two million American schoolchildren are vaccinated against polio in the largest medical experiment in the nation's history.

1962

The Migrant Health Act provides support for clinics for agricultural migrant workers.

1977

Smallpox is eradicated worldwide.

1982

The term "AIDS" (acquired immune deficiency syndrome) is used for the first time. The same year, the Gay Men Health Crisis (GMHC) is founded to help combat the disease, educate the public, and keep HIV (human immunodeficiency virus that causes AIDS) a national and local priority.

2001

In the aftermath of the terrorist attacks of September 11, health officials release a draft of the proposed Model State Emergency Health Powers Act. The act gives states greater powers to quarantine people in the event of a bioterrorist attack involving a lethal germ such as smallpox. Quarantinable diseases include cholera, diphtheria, infectious tuberculosis, plague, yellow fever, and viral hemorrhagic fevers such as Ebola.

2002

Office of Public Health Emergency Preparedness is created to coordinate efforts against bioterrorism and other emergency health threats.

2005

Hurricane Katrina destroys 80 percent of Louisiana's health-care centers and destroys all of New Orleans' health-care system and infrastructure.

2007

The Robert Wood Johnson Foundation announces $500 million pledge to fight childhood obesity.

Organizations to Contact

The editors have compiled the following list of organizations concerned with the issues debated in this book. The descriptions are derived from materials provided by the organizations. All have publications or information available for interested readers. The list was compiled on the date of publication of the present volume; the information provided here may change. Be aware that many organizations take several weeks or longer to respond to inquiries, so allow as much time as possible.

National Institutes of Health (NIH)
9000 Rockville Pike, Bethesda, MD   20892
(301) 496-4000
e-mail: NIHinfo@od.nih.gov
Web site: www.nih.gov

Founded in 1887, the National Institutes of Health is one of the world's foremost medical research centers, and the federal focal point for medical research in the United States. The NIH, comprising twenty-seven separate institutes and centers, is one of eight health agencies of the Public Health Service which, in turn, is part of the U.S. Department of Health and Human Services.

Centers of Disease Control and Prevention (CDC)
1600 Clifton Rd., Atlanta, GA   30333
(800) 311-3435
e-mail: inquiry@cdc.gov
Web site: www.cdc.gov

The CDC is the main government organization that monitors diseases and threats to the nation's health and advises the public on disease prevention at home, in the workplace, and elsewhere. One of the key tasks of the CDC is to prepare the nation for an epidemic or bioterrorist attack.

U.S. Environmental Protection Agency (EPA)
Ariel Rios Building, 1200 Pennsylvania Avenue NW
Washington, DC 20460
Web site: www.epa.gov

Established in 1970, the EPA is the federal agency whose mission is to protect human health and the environment. The EPA works for a cleaner, healthier environment by developing and enforcing regulations that implement environmental laws enacted by Congress. It sets national standards for a variety of environmental programs and issues (such as emissions) and issues sanctions to help states and tribes in reaching the desired levels of environmental quality.

U.S. Food and Drug Administration (FDA)
5600 Fishers Lane, Rockville, MD 20857-0001
(888) INFO-FDA
Web site: www.fda.gov

The FDA is the main government organization that monitors the safety of the nation's food and drugs. Decisions made by the FDA affect every American every day. Among other things, the FDA ensures that foods are safe, wholesome, and truthfully labeled, that drugs and vaccines are safe, that blood for transfusions is safe and in adequate supply, that medical devices are safe and effective, and that cosmetics are safe to use.

For Further Research

Books

Arthur Allen. *Vaccine: The Controversial Story of Medicine's Greatest Lifesaver.* New York: W.W. Norton, 2007.

Karen Buhler-Wilkerson. *No Place Like Home: A History of Nursing and Home Care in the United States.* Baltimore: Johns Hopkins University Press, 2003.

Daniel Eli Burnstein. *Next to Godliness: Confronting Dirt and Despair in Progressive Era New York City.* Urbana and Chicago: University of Illinois Press, 2006.

Karen Clay and Werner Troesken. *Deprivation and Disease in Early Twentieth-Century America.* Washington, DC: National Bureau of Economic Research, 2006.

James Keith Colgrove. *State of Immunity: The Politics of Vaccination in Twentieth-Century America.* Berkeley: University of California Press, 2006.

Sharron Dalton. *Our Overweight Children: What Parents, Schools, and Communities Can Do to Control the Fatness Epidemic.* Berkeley: University of California Press, 2004.

John Duffy. *The Sanitarians: A History of American Public Health.* Urbana and Chicago: University of Illinois Press, 1990.

Gerard T. Koeppel. *Water for Gotham: A History.* Princeton, NJ: Princeton University Press, 2000.

Alan M. Kraut. *Goldberger's War: The Life and Work of a Public Health Crusader.* New York: Hill & Wang, 2003.

Judith Walzer Leavitt. *The Healthiest City: Milwaukee and the Politics of Health Reform.* Princeton, NJ: Princeton University Press, 1992.

————. *Typhoid Mary: Captive to the Public's Health*. Boston: Beacon, 1996.

Howard Markel. *When Germs Travel: Six Major Epidemics That Have Invaded America Since 1900 and the Fears They Have Unleashed*. New York: Pantheon, 2004.

Fitzhugh Mullan. *Plagues and Politics: The Story of the United States Public Health Service*. New York: Basic, 1989.

Mazyck Ravenel, M.D., ed. *A Half Century of Public Health. Jubilee Historical Volume of the American Public Health Association*. New York: American Public Health Association, 1921.

Robert Rinsky, ed. *Public Health Reports Historical Collection, 1878–2005*. Washington, DC: Association of Schools of Public Health, 2006.

Charles Rosenberg. *The Cholera Years: The United States in 1832, 1849, and 1866*. Chicago and London: The University of Chicago Press, 1987.

David Rosner. *Are We Ready? Public Health Since 9/11*. Berkeley: University of California Press, Milbank Memorial Fund, 2006.

————. *Hives of Sickness: Public Health and Epidemics in New York City*. New Brunswick, NJ: Rutgers University Press, 1995.

Joel A. Tarr. *The Search for the Ultimate Sink: Urban Pollution in Historical Perspective*. Akron, OH: University of Akron Press, 1996.

Nancy Tomes. *The Gospel of Germs: Men, Women, and the Microbes in American Life*. Cambridge, MA: Harvard University Press, 1998.

Bernard J. Turnock. *Public Health: What It Is and How It Works*. New York: Jones & Bartlett, 2004.

John Ward and Christian Warren. *Silent Victories: The History and Practice of Public Health in Twentieth-Century America*. New York: Oxford University Press, 2007.

John H. Warner and Janet A. Tighe, eds. *Major Problems in the History of American Medicine and Public Health: Documents and Essays*. Boston: Houghton Mifflin, 2001.

Periodicals

Chris L. Barrett, Stephen G. Eubank, and James P. Smith. "If Smallpox Strikes Portland . . ." *Scientific American*, March 2005, pp. 54–61.

Jia-Rui Chong. "U.S. Issues Guidelines for Flu Crisis," *Los Angeles Times*, February 2, 2007.

W. Wayt Gibbs. "Obesity: An Overblown Epidemic," *Scientific American*, June 2005.

Bernadine Healy. "One Puff Above the Limit," *U.S. News & World Report*, February 12, 2007, p. 83.

Derrick Z. Jackson. "Diabetes: The Silent Killer Among Us," *Boston Globe*, September 30, 2006, p. A11.

Harold Jaffe. "Whatever Happened to the U.S. AIDS Epidemic?" *Science*, August 27, 2004, pp. 1243–44.

Ivan Oransky. "Medical Nihilism and the HPV Vaccine," *Boston Globe*, March 4, 2007, p. E9.

Rita Rubin. "Vaccines: Mandate or Choice?" *USA Today*, February 8, 2007, p. D6.

Stephanie Storm. "$500 Million Pledged to Fight Childhood Obesity," *New York Times*, April 4, 2007.

Marion Warwick. "Bioterrorism and the Public Health," *Journal of Homeland Security*, July 2002.

Matthew K. Wynia and Lawrence O. Gostin. "Ethical Challenges in Preparing for Bioterrorism: Barriers Within the Health Care System," *American Journal of Public Health*, July 2004.

Internet Sources

The American Experience. "Influenza 1918," www.pbs.org/wgbh/amex/influenza.

Centers for Disease Control and Prevention. "Ten Great Public Health Achievements in the 20th Century," www.cdc.gov/oc/oc/media/tengpha.htm.

Public Health Service (PHS). "History of the Commissioned Corps," www.usphs.gov/html/history.html.

Public Health Service (PHS), Office of the Public Health Service Historian, http://lhncbc.nlm.nih.gov/apdb/phsHistory.

Index